More Moments in Time

# More Moments in Time

## IMAGES OF EXEMPLARY NURSING

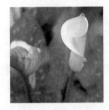

Beth Perry RN, PhD

**AU** PRESS

© 2009
BETH PERRY

Published by AU Press,
Athabasca University
1200, 10011-109 Street
Edmonton AB
T5J 3S8

**Library and Archives Canada Cataloguing in Publication**

Perry, Beth, 1957–
More moments in time : images of exemplary nursing / Beth Perry.

Includes bibliographical references.
ISBN 978-1-897425-51-0
Also available in PDF format
ISBN 978-1-897425-52-7

1. Cancer--Nursing. 2. Nursing. I. Title. II. Title: Images of exemplary nursing.

RC266.P47 2009          616.99'40231          C2009-901822-5

Printed and bound in Canada by Marquis Book Printing
Cover design by Helen Adhikari
Book layout and design by Natalie Olsen

## ACKNOWLEDGEMENTS

Photographic Images: Otto F. Mahler

Stories: The outstanding nurses who generously gave of their time and emotional energy to help me explore exemplary nursing care.

Research Funding: Social Sciences and Humanities Research Council of Canada (SSHRC)

# CONTENTS

# *preface*

## SITUATING EXEMPLARY NURSING
## IN HEALTH CARE TODAY

Since 1998, when the first version of this book, *Moments in Time:*
*Images of Exemplary Nursing Care*, was published by the Canadian
Nurses Association, Canadian health care has changed. Multiple,
potentially interrelated factors challenge Canadian nurses today.
These include personnel shortages, escalating costs and spending,
advances in technology, aging population and longer life expectancy,
increasing cultural diversity, new diseases, growing rates of chronic
diseases, shortened hospital stays, and profound ethical and moral
dilemmas. Challenges often lead to changes such as health care system
reform, evolving scope of practice with new advanced nursing prac-
tice roles, an increased 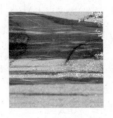 emphasis on the inter-
disciplinary team, and new approaches to health
care such as population health, integrated health
care delivery, and dis- ease management.[1] Some
argue that such changes threaten our public health
care system and the fun- damentals of universality,
comprehensiveness, accessibility, portability, and public administration. Others contend that these changes have resulted in poor practice
environments and unsatisfactory working conditions for health care
workers, especially nurses. Many question whether we can afford, or

even expect, exemplary care in a health care system that has become so complex and burdened.

Beginning with my doctoral research almost 20 years ago, I have been intrigued with what makes some clinical nurses exemplary. I defined exemplary nurses as those you would choose to have care for you or a family member. Clinical nurses (also called bedside or front line nurses) are those who spend the majority of their work time relating directly with patients.* I believe that clinical nurses are the foundation of the health care system. We simply cannot have exemplary health care without exemplary clinical nurses. Research aimed at learning more about the actions and attitudes of exemplary clinical nurses, and the effects of these on patients and on the nurses themselves, became the foundation of my program of nursing research.

## EXEMPLARY NURSES AND CAREER SATISFACTION

The findings from my initial research study on the actions, and effects of the actions, of exemplary nurses are reported in this book. Since the original project, I have completed several follow-up studies on related themes. For example, as I continued to study exemplary nurses, I discovered that they had one important commonality; they all commented often that they "loved their work." Exemplary nurses reported career satisfaction that seemed, at least in part, to motivate them to continue to provide high quality patient care.

To learn more about this possible link between career satisfaction and quality of care, I launched an international study focused on professional fulfillment in the work lives of registered nurses (RNs). I found that exemplary nurses who claimed they were satisfied with their career choices also knew their core values and believed they were able to enact these values in their workplace.[2] Their core values included altruism, caring, compassion, and a desire to make a difference. One

---

* I have chosen to use the term "patients" but I acknowledge that this group may be referred to in some health care venues as residents or clients. Their family and friends are also subsumed into the term.

important way exemplary nurses were able to make a difference for their patients was by establishing a connection with them and with their family members. These nurses found making and maintaining the connections very satisfying. When the nurses that I studied were able to provide high quality care that patients found helpful, they felt very fulfilled and found meaning in their work. Living their values, connecting with patients, and finding meaning in their work through making a difference established a cycle which propelled the exemplary nurses to continue to care in an exemplary way.[3] Career satisfaction and high quality care were the remarkable results.

A framework for career satisfaction in nursing illustrates the possible relationship between these elements and the living out of core values.[4] The dominant feature of this model is the cyclical nature of the positive caregiving experience. That is, as nurses enact their values in the workplace, connect in a meaningful way with their patients, and make a positive difference, they may realize that they become even better nurses by doing their work well and are thus motivated to continue. It is doubtful that career satisfaction in nursing is as linear as this model suggests, but it does illustrate the strong relationship between several elements identified.

When health care administrators, government officials, other stakeholders, and even nurses themselves question whether we can afford to provide high quality nursing care in these turbulent times, I say we cannot afford not to. It is in providing exemplary nursing care that nurses make a difference to patients and find meaning in their work. When nurses are professionally fulfilled, they continue to care at a high level. The resulting exemplary nursing care is not only good for the patients, it is good for the nurses too.

Another interesting finding that I am currently exploring is that the exemplary nurses I have studied very rarely report experiencing compassion fatigue (CF). Compassion fatigue is defined by LaRowe as a "heavy heart, a debilitating weariness brought about by repetitive, empathic responses to the pain and suffering of others."[5] Compassion fatigue is a term sometimes confused with burnout although the two are quite different. Schwam says that, unlike burnout which results from the stress in one's work setting that can be reversed by a vacation or a change in setting, CF is often more insidious with long-term consequences that are difficult to reverse.[6]

With a current research project, I aim to find out what it is about exemplary nurses that helps them avoid the personally and professionally devastating experience of CF. I hope that the findings of this study will have practical implications for nurse recruitment, retention, and professional well-being, if I am able to discover interventions and strategies exemplary nurses use to avoid CF.

### TIME TO CARE

A common complaint today among front line caregivers, including nurses, is that they do not have time to establish meaningful, caring, and potentially transforming relationships with their patients. The good news is that exemplary nursing care is not necessarily any more time consuming or expensive to provide than poor quality care. Admittedly, nurses are extremely busy and stress levels often run very high. Nurses may feel like they cannot squeeze one more second out of their work days. Among clinical nurses in particular, a great potential exists for turmoil, stress, burnout, and CF.[7] Yet caring is fundamental to the work of most nurses. As a nurse in one study told me, "The ability to care is nursing's common thread, and when time to express caring is denied, it is a source of frustration for me."

How can nurses provide quality care that they find satisfying within the limits of today's health care reality? Jackson emphasizes the importance of here-and-now interactions, saying that instead of feeling discouraged because of time constraints, nurses should view all of their interactions as positive and potentially effective.[8] To this end, I remind nursing students and the novice nurses I teach that it does not take any longer to administer a medication with a smile on your face than it does to give the same medication with a frown. It does not take any longer to gently rub the vein you are about to use to start the intravenous than it does to beat that vein into submission. The effect of the smile and gentle approach on the patient, and ultimately also on the nurse, is positive.

Hagerty, et al. concluded that, ideally, caregivers should have as much time as possible to be with patients.[9] When time is short, however, caregivers need not feel all is lost because every encounter between a nurse and patient can be a valuable relational moment. Each caring encounter, no matter how brief, can be important to the therapeutic relationship. For a highly skilled nurse, the connection, the experience of caring and being cared about, can happen in mere moments through the right touch, word, or listening ear. Often what patients need most is something that really does not take any extra time — a nod, a compassionate glance, or a hand placed on a shoulder at just the right moment make a positive difference for a patient and, ultimately, for the nurse as well.

Brenda,[†] an OR nurse I met, gave me an example to illustrate these points. It was a note sent to her by the wife of one of her patients:

> You probably don't remember me, but I wanted to thank you for your care. My husband and I had been in a traffic accident. The police called it a "minor traffic mishap" and after being checked over at the hospital we were both sent home. I was a little shaken and bruised, but we were both pronounced "just fine." As the week progressed I had a very disturbing dream. I dreamed that my husband was in the hospital and that he was having a cardiac arrest. I stood hopelessly by watching the team try to revive him.

† The names of the nurses, patients, and family members used in this book are all fictitious.

Imagine my horror when later that week, after he was pronounced just fine and had returned home, my husband did start to experience some perplexing symptoms and, after a consult at the emergency room, was rushed into surgery for the removal of a ruptured spleen.

The time was long as I waited, pacing the hallway outside the operating room waiting for some word on how he was doing. I was haunted by the strange dream and terrified that my husband was not going to make it through the procedure. Then I caught a glimpse of an OR nurse through the small window in the door that separates the operating area from the waiting room. That nurse was you. You were still in your scrubs and all I could see behind the green mask were your eyes. You must have seen the look of concern on my face. As you whisked about doing your post-op duties you lifted one hand and gave me the A-okay sign, your thumb and pointing finger forming a circle. This gesture took only a portion of one second, but it was all I needed to know he was all right. I just wanted to say thank you. That kindness meant so much to me.

———

**LITTLE MOMENTS**

A simple gesture.

Compassion offered. Peace received.

———

A bed bound patient once told me of his favorite nurse, calling her "the one who really cared." When I asked him what was different about this particular nurse, he said, "Every time she came into my room, she would give my big toe a little tweak." He perceived this small action as acknowledgement that made him feel connected to the nurse and cared about. Tweaking his toe took the nurse no extra time at all. Scott wrote that it is the human connection — that largely intangible, immeasurable, unquantifiable aspect of nursing practice — that nurses value most, and it is also the human connection that patients often need and desire.[10]

Clinical nursing is a demanding career. No one can be an exemplary clinical nurse without a very sound knowledge base and excellent psychomotor skills. But I have also observed that the way that care is provided — the attitude and aura of the nurses and their ability to convey compassion and caring — helps to make the care they provide exemplary. Having this certain attitude and air is not time consuming.

## NURSES RESPOND TO
### Moments in Time: Images of Exemplary Nursing Care

My 1998 book, *Moments in Time: Images of Exemplary Nursing Care*, was embraced by the nurses of Canada and all copies were sold. For experienced nurses, the stories reminded them why they chose this career and helped to reignite their passion for their profession. For the novice nurse and the nurse educator, the book was a teaching tool because it modeled effective nursing care strategies and attitudes. Additionally, nurse educators have suggested that this book could be used in first year undergraduate nursing courses on professionalism, communication, or socialization. Others have commented that it could be an exemplar of qualitative research for graduate health care courses. Instructors in nursing attendant and personal health care aide programs have suggested that the stories in the book could help to teach the enigmatic skill of caring. Other health care professionals, including pastoral care workers, rehabilitation therapists, and volunteers, have also read and valued this book and asked for more. Some have commented that the stories and analysis in this publication helped to differentiate nursing from medicine and, in doing so, helped us toward a definition of nursing. As another consequence of the book's success, I gave over 30 keynote presentations at national and international nursing conferences.

Ongoing requests for a reprinting or a new edition of the original book ultimately resulted in the publication of the book you are now reading. I hope that this updated version will contribute to scholarship in the field of nursing and to health care in general.

The lessons in this book speak of values and actions that lead not just nurses and other health care providers, but all humans, to become better. Readers of *Moments in Time* with no professional connection to health care told me, "I'm not a nurse but what you found applies to all of us," and "I felt so good after reading your book, it made me want to go out and treat my fellow man better."

For all those who have asked, I hope you enjoy this revised and updated version, *More Moments in Time: Images of Exemplary Nursing*. To the original stories and analysis, several new components are added. The preface situates exemplary nursing care in the context of the health care environment of 2009. It also features a discussion of findings of additional research on career satisfaction in exemplary nurses that arose from the original study.

Chapter 2 furthers my self-story, the multi-layered landscape of the researcher (who in qualitative research is the instrument of data collection and analysis). Since writing the original book, I have had many personal and professional experiences that have shaped what I see, believe, and know about exemplary nursing care. The assumption is that you cannot recognize what you, yourself, have not known. I hope that the additions to the section "My Memories" will give readers an insight into these influences on my research.

I have updated the citations of scholarly literature that support and enhance understanding of points made in the book. In 1998, *Moments in Time* was considered cutting edge because there were very few phenomenological nursing studies of exemplary nursing care.[‡]

---

‡ Phenomenology/phenomenological/hermeneutic phenomenology — a qualitative research tradition that focuses on the lived experience of humans. Phenomenology becomes hermeneutical when its method is taken to be interpretive (see the Appendix for more details).

Such approaches were new to the landscape of nursing. Now a new generation of nurse researchers have used phenomenology to try to capture and share the essence of nursing practice. References throughout this revised edition cite these recent studies. Other topic areas in the book, such as humour, silence, touch, and connection, have also benefited from newer research so I have cited these sources.

As I presented my research findings to audiences at conferences and workshops, I sought ways to help convey the tacit, unspoken aspects of the intense human to human interaction that often occurred in exemplary nursing situations. To do so, I turned to writing poems that help to capture the essence of an interaction in very few words. (My process is explained in detail in the Appendix.) I also experimented with using photographic images during presentations to help evoke the emotion of the story being told. Many people noted that these images gave voice to the people in the stories, again without words, which can sometimes be limiting and imposing. I have included an example of an image used to help convey the deeper meaning of the theme at the beginning of each chapter in this new edition. The poems in which I attempt to capture the essence of the nurse-patient interactions in a phenomenological sense are placed throughout the revised book.

Finally, an Appendix has been added for those who are interested in the research design and the methodology used in the study which forms the foundation of this book. Beginning with a brief exploration of the nature of qualitative inquiry, a case is made for its use in nursing investigations that focus on human experience. The methodology used in the study, hermeneutic phenomenology, is explained. Specifics about the study participants, approaches to data collection, and methods of data analysis are described. Techniques used to maintain data trustworthiness, assumptions made, delimitations and limitations of the study, and ethical considerations are included.

To those who read the original book and provided me with helpful feedback and critique, thank you. Many said that it reawakened in them their own lived experience as nurses and caregivers. I have not given a presentation based on this research without several people approaching me afterward to tell me *their* stories. To me, this is the true test of phenomenology. The research sparked memories of your own lived experiences as exemplary nurses, or exemplary human beings. Thank you all for the work you do, and that you will continue to do.

You do work wonders.


Beth Perry
Edmonton, Canada
February, 2009

# chapter one

## THE POWER AND PROMISE
## OF EXEMPLARY NURSING CARE

Within most disciplines there are those who are recognized by their colleagues as being exceptionally competent practitioners. These people are sometimes called "expert," "unusually competent," or "extraordinary." Their commonality is that they do their work in a remarkable way, and their actions and interpersonal interactions are regarded by others as highly successful.

This book is based on the findings of a 1998 study of the beliefs, actions, and interactions of a group of unusually competent oncology nurses. The investigation centered on the broad question: What is the nature of exemplary 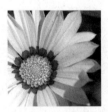 nursing practice? The nurses I studied were chosen by peer nomination. These were the nurses their peers would choose to have care for them if they were diagnosed with cancer. Data were gathered through observation, interview, and narrative exchange. The moments that appear on the pages of this book are the exemplary nurses' stories and excerpts from field notes I made during observations of their work (see Appendix).

Clinical nurses, nurse educators, nurse researchers, and nurse administrators may find this book of value. In a broad sense, the images of exemplary nursing presented here could also have meaning for practitioners and theoreticians employed in human service fields other than nursing. In fact, the issues addressed are those basic to the experience of being human: life, death, and in between, caring. For this reason, the stories and poems that are the centerpiece of this work have potential to touch all persons.

### SIGNIFICANCE FOR NURSES

Clinical nurses often work in isolation. Reading about the practice of others can be a method of learning alternative approaches to practice. In this way, the examples in this book may serve as models for beginning nurses, helping them learn both the tangible and the less tangible components of excellent practice.

Some of the descriptions provided are examples of how exemplary nurses achieve their levels of competence. From these, nurse educators can draw ideas to increase the effectiveness of their teaching. There are also worthy insights in this book for nurse educators concerned with providing continuing education for those who are already excellent practitioners.

For nurse researchers, this book is a source of unanswered questions. I anticipate that nurse researchers may use the descriptions, the questions raised, and the insights articulated, to stimulate their ideas and hypotheses for future research. One of the data collection strategies I used in this study, narrative exchange, I developed for this purpose. Certain data analysis approaches, including poetic interpretation and the use of images to convey the tacit and non-verbal, may be of interest to nurse researchers seeking innovative data collection and analysis strategies for qualitative research.

Nurse administrators may use the findings presented in several ways. For example, it may benefit them to have descriptions of the more intangible and immeasurable aspects of nursing practice. This information should be useful to administrators as they attempt to define and defend the distinctive role that nursing has in the delivery of health care.

## SIGNIFICANCE FOR OTHERS

In one sense, this book describes aspects of a greater search for what it means to be human. As we search for meaning in our experience, and in the experience of others, we gain a fuller grasp of what it means to live in this world. Van Manen claims that, through such an exploration, we "become more fully aware of who we are."[11] Those whose responsibility it is to provide service to others may find they are better able to achieve their goals if they first have a greater understanding of themselves. This work contains guidance for those who seek to become exceptional no matter what their field of service.

The nature of nursing is such that each day practitioners face some of the most fundamental and poignant issues confronting humanity. Understanding the beliefs of exceptional nurses may also illuminate our broader understanding of such issues. Ellis and Flaherty contend that "little has been done to unravel the complex manner in which emotion, cognition, and the lived body intertwine."[12] I believe that this work begins to unravel the mystery.

## DISCOVERING MEANINGS

To come to the understandings presented, the data were analyzed in several ways. The initial analysis was done by the study participants, the nurses who provided it voluntarily as they shared their narrative accounts and conversed with me.

Weaving the nurses' narratives and comments with field notes and quotations from related literature provided additional perspectives. These elements were arranged in themes. The integration of the literature into the description of the themes provided an exploration consistent with a hermeneutic phenomenological approach. Poetic interpretations were also incorporated into the hermeneutic analysis. Hopefully, these poems provide both a summary of veiled meanings contained in the narratives, comments, and observations and a further analysis. In some ways, poems expose the tacit and communicate the emotion of the situation described, leaving the reader with a greater understanding of the experience.

The final analysis is left to the readers to form their own insights regarding exceptional nursing practice. Much of the data is presented in verbatim form to facilitate this personal analysis.

In summary, this book attempts to convey research findings that include the context and humanness of the experience of exemplary nursing care. I hope what you, the reader, will take away from reading *More Moments in Time: Images of Exemplary Nursing* is a sense that you can be exemplary; that you can do small things with a sincere heart that will realistically change the world of people who need care; and that, even with the limits of the current health care environment, you can make a difference for the vulnerable people you care for.

### THE ORGANIZATION OF THIS BOOK

After I introduce the concept of exemplary nursing care in chapter 1, the second chapter sets the contextual basis for the book. I share my most vivid memories of oncology nursing in an attempt to establish a landscape against which a description and discussion of exemplary practice can be placed. In these memories I also introduce myself to you, exposing some of my values and possible biases, allowing you to decide how I may have influenced what appears on these pages. I have added relevant personal reflections on moments that have occurred since the book was first published. To expand the context for the book, I have also included a brief review of literature on the nature of oncology nursing plus comments from some of the exceptional nurses on their views of that subject.

Chapters 3, 4, and 5 each centre on a specific theme that I discovered in my study of exemplary nurses. In these three chapters, stories, quotations, observational accounts, relevant literature, and poetic analysis are used to illustrate each of the three themes: the dialogue of silence, mutual touch, and sharing the lighter side of life.

In Chapter 6 I describe the essence of the experience of exemplary nursing practice, joint transcendence. Other effects of the actions and interactions discussed in the sixth chapter include connecting and affirming the value of the patient and the nurse. Again, the nurses' stories and my poems are featured.

Major insights and implications for clinical nurses, nurse educators, nurse researchers, nurse administrators, and human services workers are presented in the final chapter.

The Appendix provides a summary of the research design and methodology used in the research that is the foundation for this book. This includes a description of ethical considerations, participants, limitations, and other elements of research design that might be of interest to readers.

For many years scholars have asked and attempted to address the question: What is nursing? Though I have tried to answer it here, many still search for a more complete appreciation. My hope is that those who choose to read this book will emerge with enhanced understanding of the power and promise of exemplary nursing care and at least a partial answer to one of the toughest questions I know.

—

### I AM YOUR NURSE

I am your nurse.
I ease your pain.
I bathe your skin.
I make your bed.
I help you dress.
I meet your needs.
You heal me.

I am your nurse.
I feed you meals.
I give you rest.
I tend your wounds.
I sense your suffering.
I answer your questions.
You teach me.

I am your nurse.
I know your pain.
I share your loneliness.
I feel your despair.
I taste your joy.
I sense your spirit.
You touch my soul.

And sometimes,
for just a moment,
I am you,
and you are me,
and we are one.

Together,
we go beyond the limits
of ordinary experience,
to live the extraordinary.

——

# *chapter two*

## THE MULTI-LAYERED
## LANDSCAPE

Exemplary nursing practice is complex. Part of the complexity comes from the intricate and multi-faceted nature of the context in which nursing occurs. This context or landscape needs to be articulated so that descriptions of exceptional nursing practice can be clearly viewed. As a preamble, a brief review of the literature on the nature of oncology nursing is presented. Statements from conversations with unusually competent nurses are highlighted in a discussion of some particular features of cancer, the disease of primary interest to oncology nurses.

This landscape also includes a collection of my memories, stories from my experience as an 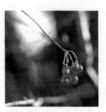 oncology nurse, educator, and researcher. By shar- ing these vignettes, I hope to convey something of my values, beliefs, and possible biases. Encour- aging readers to incorpo- rate an understanding of my experiences into their own stock of knowledge will increase their general understanding of me, of oncology nursing, and ultimately of exem- plary nursing practice.

The first part of the "My Memories" section of this chapter features stories from my early experience as newly graduated oncology nurse. For the second edition of this book, I have updated my self-story. It now includes personal experiences that have occurred during the ten years since the first edition of this book was published. These reflections may be relevant to readers who seek to understand how the researcher, as an instrument of data collection and analysis, filters what is observed and how it is interpreted.

### CARING FOR PEOPLE WITH CANCER

Nursing has been acknowledged in the literature as both a demanding and rewarding profession.[13,14] An essential feature of nursing is that it is an experience lived between human beings, primarily between patients and nurses. A therapeutic, goal-oriented process, nursing service is directed at meeting patient needs. These needs may be physical, psychological, intellectual, or spiritual in nature and will differ with varying health problems.

Nurses often hold the fragility of human life in their hands as part of their everyday work life. Routinely administering complex treatments that allow for a very small margin of error can be stressful. The knowledge explosion in health care has resulted in the increased use of technology and has further complicated treatment protocols. Among the responsibilities assumed by nurses are the promotion and restoration of health, prevention of illness, attainment of a peaceful death, and maintenance of a therapeutic environment in which these goals may be achieved.

As a first line of defense and advocacy for the patient, the nurse is in a position of privilege and responsibility. This responsibility necessitates establishing and maintaining relationships with multiple professional groups. Nurses working a variety of shifts provide nursing services to patients 24 hours a day. These considerations can make nursing physically and emotionally exhausting. Fagin and Diers assert that,

Nursing is a metaphor for intimacy. Nurses are involved in the most private aspects of people's lives and they cannot hide behind technology or a veil of omniscience as other practitioners...in hospitals do. Nurses do for others publicly what healthier persons do for themselves behind closed doors. Nurses are there to hear secrets, especially the ones born of vulnerability.[15]

Benner and Wrubel contend that those who choose to be nurses can expect frustration, despair, highs, lows, and defeats often enough to remain humble.[16] Yet, as Peplau concluded over a century earlier, nursing can be a maturing force and an educative instrument.[17] Mallison expresses it this way:

If you keep working at it, learning from it...gradually you realize your palette is filling up with colors. You see more shades of meaning. You realize you are well on your way to creating a work of art, maybe even a masterpiece.[18]

Oncology (cancer) nursing is a specific form of medical-surgical nursing. Nurses who specialize in oncology provide nursing services to people who have cancer throughout the stages of the disease. This specialty is unique for many reasons.

First, cancer is a very common and serious disease. In 2004, cancer was the leading cause of death for Canadians aged 35 to 64 years and the second leading cause of death for most other age groups.[19] The prevalence of cancer means that most oncology nurses have had a personal association with the disease through family or friends. Some nurses have been treated for cancer themselves.

Second, the treatment of cancer is usually a lengthy process, often causing disruption in the work and family life of the patient. These disruptions, combined with the plaguing side effects of the therapies, place demands on the patient, the patient's family, and the caregivers.

Highfield writes,

> A diagnosis of cancer often provokes a crisis of mean-
> ing. Personal relationships may be burdened with an
> uncertain future. Formerly effective coping strategies
> seem inadequate...there is a rising sense of aloneness.
> In short, a spiritual crisis is created.[20]

Third, the guilt associated with having cancer adds to the suffering
of the patients and their families. Julie, one of the exemplary nurses,
phrased it like this:

> Though the etiologies of many cancers are unproven,
> a diagnosis of cancer is often accompanied by guilt.
> There is a whole school of thought out there that proj-
> ects to the vulnerable, grieving, cancer patient that this
> whole disease is their fault. Comments like, "You can
> fight this thing," or "With the proper attitude it can
> be overcome," make them feel responsible both for get-
> ting sick and for getting well. There probably is some-
> one somewhere who drank a herbal tea, prayed in a
> certain position, ate peach pits, or laughed themselves
> into being reportedly free of cancer. But it makes the
> remaining millions feel abjectly guilty, as if they have
> done something wrong.

Fourth, cancer is culturally among the most dreaded diseases. One of
the most frightening sentences a person might hear is, "You have cancer." These words bring a chill to the heart. Although some progress
has been made in treating cancer, recovery can be long and painful
and many people do not survive. Its chronicity and close association
with death and suffering make it a somewhat taboo topic in our society. According to Benner and Wrubel,

In society the disease cancer appears to have become the metaphor for the deepest fears held about the inevitable disintegration and decay of the body. Cancer is the disease which attacks the body organs about which greatest ambivalences are felt, those of sexuality, reproduction, and excretion. The society "battle" against cancer is then seen as the struggle to resist acceptance of the inevitability in life of death, decay, and decomposition.[21]

Glaser and Strauss, after extensive study of cancer care settings, conclude that the illness is often more difficult for caregivers and survivors than for patients.[22] Benner and Wrubel agree that providing nursing service for cancer patients is especially challenging because nurses need to "adopt ingenious strategies for providing comfort, nutrition, social support, rest, and activity in the midst of demanding treatment regimes and a debilitating disease."[23]

Julie, an exemplary nurse I studied, summarized her view of the devastating nature of cancer in the following comment:

We must realize that cancer is relentless and shows absolutely no respect for its host. Cancer writes its own rules. It teases, in fact, each remission gives a little taste of hope for normalcy. Then, there is the emotional murder of recurrence, just to reassure patients that they are at the mercy of this monster and needn't begin to think otherwise.

## MY MEMORIES

We are all a collection of the significant moments of our individual lives, our moments in time. Julie said,

> If life could be distilled down to one hour in time, that hour would include a cluster of significant moments. A moment is that which recurs when needed; it is that recurrence which magnifies the significance. These moments fill our memory banks. They are our resource files, our warm fuzzies, the emotional adhesive that holds us together. They are us.

I believe that my "moments in time" have a place in this work. I want to share something of myself with you, and I feel these memories of my life as a clinical nurse are one way to accomplish this. By including these stories, I am not claiming that I am — or was — an exceptional practitioner. My purpose instead is to provide a small number of my more potent memories from my experiences, thereby imparting some understanding of this world of cancer care, and of me.

## The Day I Became a Nurse

*She was so ill. She was bleeding to death in front of my eyes, and there was little that I, or anyone, could do. As I helped her back to bed, her three beautiful teenage sons pressed closer to the wall and watched in horror. Not knowing how to help her, I sat down on her bed and took her hand tightly in mine. Putting aside all thoughts of the half dozen other patients who needed me, I let my energy flow into her. As silent seconds passed, I felt some of her spirit pour into me. At that moment I was changed. At that moment I became a nurse.*

## The Bald Man with the Big Laugh

*I had just been appointed chemotherapy nurse, a position I assumed with much pride and enthusiasm. The emphasis of my duties would now be on something I really enjoyed doing: teaching the patients about the drugs they were to receive.*

*As with any new responsibility, there was a certain amount of anxiety at first, and I was shaking a little as I approached Mr. and Mrs. Zimmerman to teach them about Mr. Zimmerman's chemotherapy. However, I was determined to do well, and I had a sophisticated teaching plan—complete with objectives—in hand. Sitting down, I launched into my lecture about the side effects of the drug he was to receive—the major one in his case being anticipated hair loss. At one point in my monologue, I realized that both Mr. and Mrs. Zimmerman were looking at me with some amusement. Pausing long enough to assess the situation, I realized to my embarrassment that Mr. Zimmerman was already totally bald—and had been for many years as a result of natural causes. I stopped speaking, stammered a little, and then we all burst into a cleansing round of laughter—laughter that swelled until the tears came.*

## On Melting Anger

*She was such a gruff woman. My most vivid memories of her revolve around her sitting upright in her bed issuing caustic commands to her family members and caregivers. Being a novice nurse who was eager to please, I was succulent prey for her and she was crude, harsh, and cutting in her demands of me. "Move that water jug," "Fluff my pillow," "Bring me juice," she would snap. Often I was afraid to answer her call bell and face her anger. Yet as the days went on, I started to like her. I looked forward to seeing her and being her nurse.*

*One day in response to her demand that I "help her out of bed, NOW," I put my arm around her shoulders to offer her support. "What are you doing?" she barked. As our eyes met, I said, "I'm just trying to help you; I want you to be as comfortable as possible, and I don't want you to fall and*

31

*hurt yourself." She muttered a muted "oh" but, at the same time, as I held her emaciated frame tightly, I felt some of her muscles relax just a little and I knew that I had touched her with my touch.*

## A Good Death

*The warm amber glow of a candle filters through the quiet air. In the bed covered with a patchwork quilt that she has made, a middle-aged woman breaths shallow, erratic last breaths. Her husband of a quarter century sits at her side brushing her cheeks with his stocky fingers and with occasional soft kisses. Although she is unable to talk, he tells her how much their life together has meant to him and how much he will miss her. As her breathing ceases, he gives her a final kiss and turns to me. Freely, I open my arms and my heart to him in his grief. I leave them alone for a moment to say goodbye. As I go, he says, "Thank you." I smile inside, feeling privileged to have shared in the final moments of their life together.*

## Mama Goes to Heaven

*The soft strains of music touch me as I enter her room. Around the bed, her eight children stand hand in hand. My patient is a recently immigrated Italian woman of 60 years. Her life is nearly ended, and pain remains her greatest adversary. No amount of analgesic has soothed the relentless agony. Quietly, her family begins to work magic. As they sing softly in their native tongue, my patient dozes in peace. They take turns—sometimes singing joyously in unison; other times, a sweet, sad, solo voice is heard. As they sing, she slowly slips away. They each say goodbye to their "Mama" and then move on to live the rest of their now more precious lives. After they have gone, I say my own farewell to this brave lady, and I feel honored to have helped escort her to peaceful rest.*

## Learning the Value of Honesty

*Being so young, she quickly became everyone's favorite patient. As I enter her room, she sits on her bed cross-legged, neon clad, and hugging a huge stuffed elephant. For several seconds I stare at her, struck again by the incongruence of the childlike face so clouded by the haggard expression of one who has experienced the stress of chronic terminal illness. As I sit down beside this child, she looks at me and asks with penetrating frankness, "Am I going to die?" In the timeless seconds that follow, my mind races, searching frantically for an answer and rejecting all the possibilities. Finally, my lips open and, as honestly and gently as I can, I say "Yes." I know my eyes filled with tears first as we dissolved into one another's arms, grasping for the comfort of human touch. How utterly important she was to me at that moment, and how vital I was to her.*

## The Secret Whispers

*"I miss them so much," she sighed as I washed her back and tried to make her more comfortable. "I haven't seen my kids for nearly a month. I would give anything to give them a hug." I touched her hand and, as our eyes met, I knew I had to help her.*

*Two days later it happened. Three preschoolers climbed onto their Mom's bed and blanketed her in hugs, kisses, and cookie crumbs. It was such a joyous afternoon. As they leave her to return home, she plants a secret whisper in each small ear—a whisper of her exclusive love for each of them. Each one is her "favorite" child and always will be.*

*Later that week as we struggle to save her fragile life, she opens her dying eyes just long enough to tell me a secret. "Please let me go," she whispers, "I'm ready." As we withdraw the life-support equipment, I am overcome with feelings of peace and achievement. We have given her the greatest gifts possible for her—secret moments with her children and death with dignity.*

## Silent Music

*In report they announce that I am to give one-to-one care to a young woman with leukemia. She is distressed and agitated because of recent news that her disease is out of remission. Knowing that I will be her constant companion for the next eight hours, I try to think carefully about the approach I will take in our conversation. What should I say? How can I let her know that what she is feeling is normal? What can I do to offer her the support I know she needs?*

*As I enter her room, I am still unsure of my opening words, so I say nothing. Sitting close to her on her bed, I take her cold hand in mine. Softly stroking her forehead, I speak only with my eyes and touch. She seems relieved, and I can feel the tension ease. The silence, it appears, is a welcomed friend. It feels tranquil. Nothing is frantic; nothing needs to be said. It is as if the agony and strain have been replaced by music that we can both hear.*

## Caring On

*"Here is your patient for today." As I get off the elevator, I look up to the voice of my charge nurse. She is holding a tiny baby wrapped in a hospital blanket, and she is handing the babe to me. Involuntarily, my head is shaking no, while inside I struggle to confirm what is happening. A baby — with cancer — my patient? It just can't be.*

*But it is true. As she transfers the wee infant to my arms, I recognize the unmistakable look of the disease etched on the little face. She is swollen from the medications, and her bald head carries the bruises and scars of repeated intravenous insertions. The grey-yellow complexion of death is indisputable.*

*That intense encounter with the brutal injustice of cancer followed me throughout my career. Occasionally, I wonder how I kept going — how I kept caring. Much of my motivation came from a tiny pendant given to me by a friend. I wore it always. Once in a while, I would catch a glimpse of it in a mirror as I gave my patients care. "Live–love–laugh," was its message. Whenever I saw it, I knew I must carry on — for my sake, for the sake of that innocent child, and for the patients I was yet to meet.*

As I relive these events from my early nursing years, I recall that the anguish was often great. However, through these same experiences came a sense of achievement and the knowledge that I was making a difference in the lives of others. For me, cancer nursing was an incredible opportunity — a chance to be intimately involved with people who were entering one of the most critical times of their lives.

What a privilege it was to encounter the humanness of life as part of my everyday work life. I feel that I have been shaped by my experiences with cancer patients and their families. Seeing others bravely facing their disease, their treatments, and their uncertain futures helped me realize how precious and precarious life is. As a result of these experiences, my life became brighter and more full of texture. Personal relationships were enriched and life took on a strange combination of urgency on one hand, and relaxed animation on the other. I was inspired to laugh liberally, cry openly, care deeply, and study intently while at the same time savouring every second of each experience.

—

**NURSE TRANSFORMED**

Shaped and molded daily by
a constant stream of challenges,
you continue to evolve.

Each time you confront death,
all life becomes more treasured.

Now,
you approach life with a sense of urgency,
eagerly soaking up all of the
pleasures and pains it offers.

You want to change the world,
to make a difference in the lives of
those who need you.
But all the while
you recognize that you too must be sustained
and you receive as openly as you give.
With gratitude
you accept and welcome these changes,
and anticipate your continued transformation.

—

Nursing is very complex and multi-faceted. Our understanding of the actions and thoughts of those nurses who do it exceptionally well remains limited. However, I hope that describing the ways of those nurses who provide nursing care with unusual competence can enhance our awareness and appreciation of excellent practice and move us to a fuller understanding of what nursing is.

Following completion of my PhD and the publishing of *Moments in Time*, I continued my work as a nurse educator and researcher. I broadened the patient populations I served to include people with various diseases and conditions but maintained an intense interest in exemplary nursing care, noticing that I could not ever separate my clinician hat from my educator hat from my researcher hat. Formally, I worked in various nursing roles, conducted focused research projects, and taught different groups of students (nurses and others) but, all the while, I was watching, listening, or reading with the underlying goal of continuing to discover the fundamental elements of exemplary nursing. There is a certain mystery of exceptional nursing practice that I am not sure I will ever be able to articulate within the limitation of words. But some key experiences over the more recent years have helped shaped me and what I believe about exemplary nursing.

## Tears Fall Like Rain

*When I started sharing the research findings from the original study of exemplary nursing care at conferences and workshops, I was a little surprised at how nurses—especially front line nurses who provide direct hands on care—responded to the presentations. Almost without exception, the stories and poems from the study would move the audiences to tears. I remember one lady who, after dabbing away at her eyes during my entire presentation, finally ran out of tissues and, in a very audible blow, used the fancy white tablecloth from the conference ballroom as a hanky. This resulted in gales of laughter from the group who admitted they had thought of doing the same thing!*

*I frequently pondered why hearing about exemplary nursing touched such a raw spot in the conference attendees. At first, I was very uneasy when I saw the tears begin to flow. I even tried to "lighten up" and avoid any of the really emotive stories in my presentations. Over time, I realized that nursing is emotion. We are working with people who are often at some of the most critical and difficult moments of their lives. Exemplary nurses willingly embrace this responsibility and meet their patients where they are at. Nurses who really care invite their vulnerable patients in and offer them comfort and compassion — an island of hope. At the moments when these connections between nursing and patient occur, it may not be appropriate for the nurses to share their emotions. The nurses need, in some sense, to feel — yet not feel. My belief is that when the nurses are sitting in that conference ballroom and hearing these stories that often parallel their own past encounters with vulnerable patients, it becomes a safe place for that emotion which has been held in check to be released. Tears that fall like rain can be very healing.*

## Going it Solo

*After one presentation, a nurse approached me and said, "I need to tell you one of my stories." She did not say, " I want to tell you," she said, "I need to tell you." This reinforced for me that nursing is often a very isolated activity. We work behind closed doors and pulled curtains; very often, the nurse is the only caregiver present with a patient and family. This leaves nurses very few opportunities to share their experiences (good and bad), to debrief, to receive encouragement, or even to receive a pat on the back when they are especially successful.*

*This reflection reinforced in me the importance of finding deliberate ways, safe places, and structured activities that help nurses to talk to other nurses about their professional encounters. When I have had the chance to really listen to nurses and hear their stories, not only have they seemed relieved to be able to share their successes or burdens, I have also been affected. If educators, administrators, and nurses themselves could embrace the opportunity that exists in the sharing of stories, there could be positive ramifications for nurse well-being, staff retention, and quality of patient care. Tell your stories — they are you.*

## It's the Little Things

*After sharing the original themes and collecting new data during studies of nursing career satisfaction, it became even more obvious to me that it is the little things — the simple gestures rendered with a compassionate heart — that really make the difference between being a great nurse and being an exemplary nurse. Of course, to be great, a nurse needs a deep knowledge base and exceptional psychomotor skills — but, to be truly outstanding, a nurse needs to be attentive to the small, and at first seemingly insignificant, elements of a nurse-patient relationship. For example, a good nurse can competently initiate an intravenous (IV). An exemplary nurse would start that same IV in the same amount of time but would probably leave the patient feeling more cared about. The difference is that the exemplary nurse makes eye contact with the patient, gently rubs the vein to be punctured, and smiles warmly — genuinely — as she leaves the room. These are such small things, but they help maintain the dignity of the patient.*

*The stories in this book are rich with examples of how it was the little things that the nurse said or did that really laid the foundation for making a positive difference for the patient. I challenge the reader to keep this idea in mind and to identify these exemplary practices as the book is read.*

*As with all phenomena, there is a shadow side. It is also the smallest actions or comments that can inflict damage on the therapeutic potential of a nurse-patient relationship. Uttered thoughtlessly, the words, "There is nothing more we can do for you," or "I don't have time for you," can devastate a vulnerable patient or family. A medication handed over roughly or a bathroom door left embarrassingly open can make the difference between trust established or trust destroyed. Mother Teresa's words, "It's not the big things; it's the little things done with great love," certainly are true.*

## On Boundaries

*Exemplary nurses have confidence and self-assurance and are willing to take appropriate risks with what we have labeled "professional boundaries." Since carrying out the initial research, I have watched more exemplary nurses in action and noticed that they often stretched what some would say were the bounds of appropriate behaviour for a professional nurse. Few nurses truly come to care about their patients (and their families). This may sound like a contradiction—after all, isn't nursing really about caring? I am not sure that all nurses do allow themselves to become emotionally entwined with patients—ever. Those nurses who are exemplary however, do—at least at some level. Exemplary nurses are willing to share something of themselves with their patients and invite at least some of their patients, some of the time, into their hearts. These nurses are often, in return, changed in a positive way by such encounters. Is this blurring of professional boundaries appropriate? Often I have been challenged by those who say it is not. Yet, if you talk to exemplary nurses, they say that it is these experiences where they feel especially close to specific patients or family members that have taught them the most and that have fueled their ability to continue to care.*

## Affirmation

*We do not often stop to acknowledge success—in ourselves or in others. Yet, it is the knowledge that they have made a positive difference in the lives of patients or family members that often drives nurses to continue to care. In studies of career satisfaction in nursing, I looked for nurses who genuinely could say, "I love my work." Then I asked these nurses to tell me about the times when they knew they had made the right career choice. Without exception, these moments of professional fulfillment revolved around an experience where they had come to know they had made a difference. This understanding may have come from a patient, a visitor, a colleague, a supervisor, or from that quiet voice inside. But successfully softening the suffering of another vulnerable person facilitated a sense of career fulfillment and fuelled these nurses to continue to do their work in an exemplary way. Yet how often do we purposefully notice and acknowledge these moments, in ourselves and in others? After learning more about the importance of acknowledgment, I take the time, take the risk, and share the good things that I see. Nurses do work wonders.*

Not all of my personal experiences with nursing and nurses over the more recent years have been positive. When you have on the researcher glasses, continually seeking to understand nursing care, you cannot remove them when you are put in the role of family member. Over the past eight years, I have been the daughter with elderly parents and in-laws in health care situations. These experiences have further shaped the lenses through which I view exemplary nursing care. I have learned that I can also learn about exemplary nursing by experiencing less than stellar care. My role as a daughter wanting to ensure adequate care for the important elderly people in my life influenced my understand of nursing, especially the care of the aged. In response, I wrote the following editorial for a local radio broadcast.

## Daughter, not Nurse

*I remember reading a letter to the editor awhile ago. It began, "When my Mom entered a nursing home, I promised I would always protect her. In the end, I could not keep my promise." When I read this, I thought with some indignation, "Of course she could have protected her Mom. She just didn't try hard enough." Today I take back that judgement.*

*After journeying with my own mom and mother-in-law for nearly four years as they have lived in continuing care, I too admit I have failed to protect them. In spite of spending six to eight hours a day with them, seven days a week, 365 days a year, and in spite of hiring extra personal companion care for them for 40 hours a week, I haven't been able to protect them at this time in their lives when they are as vulnerable as small children.*

*Protect them from what you might ask? Protect them from medication not given or medications given twice; protect them from being rushed or being lectured for "bad" behaviour they can't control; protect them from harsh words uttered by staff who can't understand what they are trying to say; protect them from having things done to them that they don't want done, or from having things not done that they desperately want. I haven't protected their feelings from being hurt by uncaring comments. I haven't protected their spirits from being dashed by rough treatment or from being ignored altogether as if they are somehow invisible objects in the room as the caregivers do their tasks.*

*If children were treated as these elders are treated, their caregivers would be charged with abuse. Yet because they are old, because they are often sick, because they drool, because they slur their speech, because they wet their pants, because they can't move, or talk, or walk fast, it becomes acceptable in the eyes of society to mistreat elders in these ways.*

*Why don't more family members speak up? In my experience, they do try to advocate for their loved ones — at least when they are first admitted to continuing care facilities. But eventually it becomes too much — the constant need to be vigilant, the chronic disappointment with the care, the trust often broken. Perhaps denial and avoidance become their best modes of coping. Soon the sons and daughters visit less often and the seniors are largely abandoned to the system.*

*How can we change this situation so that elders in care facilities get the compassionate care they need and deserve? More money, more staff, and more education are not the answers. The change can only start more fundamentally with a change in attitude. We need to become a society that values and protects our elders, a society that embraces the wisdom that often comes with age, a society that cares for the most vulnerable with compassion, and a society that vows to never destroy hope in the aged.*

The secrets of being an exemplary nurse do not only apply to nurs-ing. In reality, being an excellent nurse — the nurse people would choose to have care for them if they were ill — comes down to treat-ing others as you would like to be treated. The exemplary nurse is not that much different than the exemplary store clerk, janitor, teacher, lawyer, or bus driver. My niece Sarah told me a story that really solidified this thinking for me.

## Simply Profound

Sarah was working late one night at university (she is a first year environ-mental science student). She had been working all day on a lab and was just about finished when she decided to tidy up the lab and delete some unnecessary data. You guessed it — the delete button bombed her entire lab and she had to start again. Needless to say, when she finally trudged to the bus stop that night to start her long trip home, she was tired, hungry and a little down.

Then along came her bus and a driver that would change her day. She said that, when the door of the bus opened, an unfamiliar rather elderly ("elderly" was her word — he was likely 50) male driver said with a big smile, "Well, hello, young lady. Welcome aboard. Just come on in and make yourself comfortable." Sarah said with this greeting she was already start-ing to feel a little better. She watched as this scene repeated itself at each subsequent stop with the driver greeting each new passenger heartily. Then, as they drove through the Old Strathcona area of the city, the driver made like a tour guide and boomed out "Ladies and gentlemen — you will notice that we are now entering the Old Strathcona area of Edmonton. I am sure that you will enjoy the many fine dining establishments and trendy shopping." Sarah said by this time everyone on the bus was smiling and exchanging amused glances. When an older lady with a cane made her way to the front of the bus to exit, she paused to say to the man, "In my 30 years of riding the bus, you are the best bus driver I have ever had?" To this, he replied, "I know! My wife tells me the same thing every morn-ing as I leave for work."

*Sarah said she usually reads on the bus, but on this trip she was so totally enthralled with the driver and his actions that the trip flew by and she arrived home feeling much better.*

Exemplary nursing is really, at least in part, all about being an exemplary human being. It is about making people feel welcome and comfortable, treating others as you would like to be treated, giving information if it is appropriate and people want to hear it, staying positive in a sea of negativity, having self-confidence and self-awareness, being able to accurately assess the needs of those around you and responding to these, loving your work and letting your enthusiasm show. Exemplary nursing — it's so simple; it's so profound.

# *chapter 3*

## THE DIALOGUE OF
## SILENCE

Silence: pure, precise, and — in a sense — perfect. There is little written about it. Silence is seldom a direct focus of research or conversation because silence is difficult to observe, record, and write about. A 2008 search of the literature on silence as a nursing intervention turned up only five scholarly publications on the topic.

Silence emerged repeatedly as an approach used by the exemplary nurses in my study. It is clear that the nurses often used silence during emotional or difficult patient interactions. Beyond these more extraordinary times, silence also played an important part in everyday nurse-patient encounters.

Silent moments were a part of most nurse-patient exchanges. In few day-to-day human 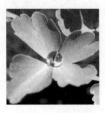 interactions is there constant, relentless verbal-ization. However, the silences that were part of these nurse-patient encounters were different from our average customary pauses. Most times these silences, or gaps in speech, were rich in non-verbal communication. Messages that were difficult or even impossible to say out loud, were sent from nurse to patient and from patient to nurse in silence. When everything that needed to be said had been said, when cultural or language barriers inhibited spoken communication, when the patient was confused, when the news was bad, when there were no "right" words, and when no words were necessary, silence was used.

There were many benefits or gifts that resulted from silence. Specifically, patients received the gift of the nurse's presence and the gift of being listened to with openness. Through providing these silent gifts, the nurses also received, making this silent dialogue beneficial to both the patient and the nurse.

It is apparent that the silence came in varying forms. For example, non-verbal messages framed in silence, silent messages encoded in words, and silent messages encoded in actions are forms of silent interplay recorded and consequently reported in this chapter. The commonality of many of the silent moments was the two-way quality. Therefore, I have called this theme the dialogue of silence.

In this chapter, I combine some of the stories written by the nurses I studied, excerpts from conversations I had with them, and my field notes. These narratives illustrate the uses, gifts, and forms of silence as well as how the nurses came to learn to use silence in patient interactions.

To provide an enhanced understanding of some of these examples, a poem that I believe exposes the nucleus or heart of the narrative is presented. I consider poetry an appropriate medium of analysis because it is a bridge between non-verbal and verbal expression and it allows for communication in a succinct and creative way. Poems potentially expose the tacit, that which is difficult to express otherwise. Together, the narratives, poems, and literature provide an understanding of how silence is used in exceptional nursing practice.

### LEARNING TO USE SILENCE

Among the exemplary nurses, there was agreement that, "you grow into the use of silence," and that it is "a very powerful and advanced skill." These nurses confirmed that they do consciously use silence in their nursing care, but this had not always been so. Many talked

about trying hard to "say the right thing" to patients and their family members early in their nursing careers. Jane, an exemplary nurse,
phrased it this way: "I found that I used to worry a lot about saying
the right thing. I have discovered that the 'right thing' often means
saying nothing at all."

Although these exemplary nurses agreed that silence is useful and
effective in conveying concern for patients and in allowing them an
opportunity to express themselves, they acknowledge that silence is
difficult to use. Lana, another of the exceptional nurses, said,

> We are a very verbal society. We talk, talk, talk. We
> hardly ever stop to really listen. We generally don't
> like silence. It is very uncomfortable, and it was for
> me, too — especially in the beginning. It's not that you
> don't want to be quiet; it's just that you can't. It's not
> natural, at least not for me anyway.

How did these nurses learn to practice silence effectively? They talked
about observing other nurses using it with their patients. "It was just
so amazing," commented Jane as she described a particular moment
when a nurse she considered very capable calmed an agitated patient
without a word by placing a quiet hand on his shoulder. Other nurses
described how they discovered the power of silence on their own,
often quite by accident. Jane told me of this experience.

> I was with this patient I didn't know very well. His
> doctor just came in his room on rounds one day and
> said, "Your cancer has spread. There is very little else
> we can do for you. It doesn't look good," and left. I was
> blown away. Because I didn't know what to say, I just sat
> down on the edge of the bed and the patient and I sat
> there looking out the window together. I just couldn't
> think of a thing to say that would counter the intensity

of what had been said, or make the patient feel any better. Finally, I just left.

A few days later that patient said, "Thanks for being there when I needed you." I learned something really important from that experience.

—

**A LESSON LEARNED**

There is a time to be silent,
and a time to speak.

The key is,
learning to tell the difference,
and having the temperance
to do what's right.

—

Part of learning to use silence is learning to hear differences in silences. Sometimes silence means that a great deal of suffering is present. Embarrassing circumstances may cause silence. Exhaustion may bring a peaceful kind of silence. Moria, one of the exceptionally competent nurses, talked of these differences when she commented, "I try to be tuned in to the variance in silent human sounds." Gauthier wrote about the variety of messages that can be communicated in silence — ranging from empathy and concern to resentment and hostility.[24] Silence becomes less threatening when this range is understood.[25] Armstrong also notes that silence has a range and, in his words, "silence can cut both ways and can leave disaster and unhappiness in its wake."[26] For example, remaining silent on errors made or failure to express a simple thank you are examples of negative silence. Silence can also be positive for the nurse-patient relationship. Armstrong gives the example of "pregnant pauses" and suggests that, when they are left to naturally unfold between patients and caregivers, these silent moments are a vehicle for facilitating rich, nonverbal communication.[27]

48

## TIMES WHEN SILENCE IS USEFUL

It appeared that the exceptional nurses used silence in a variety of situations. In particular, when there was nothing more to be said, when communicating with patients across cultures, when their patients were dying, when their patients received bad news, when their patients were psychologically or cognitively impaired, when words were unnecessary, and when there were no right words. The following sections provide examples of each of these applications.

### When it has all been said

Some relationships with patients and their families last for an extended time. In these situations the nurse may know the patient very well after journeying together through the stages in the disease trajectory. In some relationships, nothing more needs to be said, as the title of this poem suggests.

—

**THE DAY THE WORDS RAN OUT**

They have poured so freely
over the years,
like sand flowing through an hourglass.

Then one day,
like the sand,
the words just all ran out.

But don't be tempted
to turn the hourglass over,
to fill the void with endless chatter,
because no matter what you do,
the sand will never flow as smoothly again,
and we'll both just be disappointed.

—

Another exemplary nurse, Marie, told me the following story that illustrates this particular use of silence.

> Joan was my patient, but more than that we had become friends over the six years. She had come to the hospital for treatments, pain control, and now for palliative care. We had shared so much: laughter, pain, and true accomplishments. I remember how excited I felt when she was rehabilitated from major back surgery. She was able to walk again. Sure she had to use a cane, but she was travelling.... It was a miracle, and we celebrated!
>
> Now those moments were only memories as she was admitted for palliative care. I enjoyed being her nurse as we shared a lot about one another's lives. She knew of my hopes, dreams, and plans. I knew of her favorite things, her tears, and her troubles. It was Christmas, and she was assigned to me. She struggled to speak as it now required a great deal of effort. So now, I also spoke very little. She slept and dozed off frequently as the narcotics were being increased daily. When she would open her eyes, we'd smile. I remember clutching her hand just before I left my shift and holding that grip. I wished her a beautiful Christmas; peace was my greatest hope for her.
>
> I left the room. I remember wanting to go back to her and hesitating. Should I say "goodbye?" I didn't return. Over the years we had said a lot. The last day we said little and I still feel that was all that was needed. Silence speaks in gentler ways than words at times.
>
> Sometimes everything that needed to be said has already been said. If it has already been done, you have to recognize that. I had been with Joan for six years. When it

came to the end, there was nothing left to say. We had said it all. The words had just run out.

—

**THE SILENT PARTING**

We have been together for a season,
and our time has been so good.
When it's time for me to go,
just place a finger to your lips
and step away.
There are no words—no adieu,
no farewell, no goodbye,
that can say anything
that we haven't already said;
that can mean any more
than you already mean to me.

—

*When communicating across cultures*

In some cultures silence is a more accepted, and therefore a more appropriate, means of communication. During one of our conversations, Marie recalled this memory of a young boy she had cared for.

He was a young guy, a native Indian from Northern Alberta. He just didn't use many words. It wasn't his way. I knew that talking would be too much for him. It wasn't needed. When I watched his family around him, especially his Mom whom he loved very much, they just were very quiet. They just sat with him. So when I was his nurse, I tried to mirror my behaviour to theirs — although I was still me. I thought that would show respect for the ground he stood on, for his culture, his ways.... You have to be able to do that and not detract from your personality and become someone you are not. It's a real art.

Jane's story tells of a man from a different subculture of society and his silent approach to communication.

I will always remember one elderly fellow. He was a hermit; he lived in the mountains. Every day he would get up at 4:30 a.m. I would find him up in the lounge just sitting and smiling. The first time I saw him there I said, "You're up — why can't you sleep? Do you have pain? Would you like some warm milk? Shall I have the doctor order you a sleeping pill?" He just said politely, "No, no, no, no — I always get up early at home. You know the birds sing their best songs in the morning."

I just let him go with his agenda. What was I going to do — put him back to bed? He was 88 years old, and he had seen many early mornings.

I remember him because he wasn't a man of many words. I just sat with him. We both knew darn well there weren't any birds to hear, but we just sat there listening. I just sat with him.... We didn't talk much. I thought if I had been living alone all those years, I wouldn't have much to say either.

———

**REFLECTIVE SILENCE**
Meet my silence with silence.
Reflect my ways with your own.
See the me that I am,
not the me that you want me to be.
Sit with me
and let the silent notes of the birds' songs
sing to us.

———

## When the patient is dying

Patients in the final stages of their disease are often most comfortable in an environment that provides limited stimulation, including a reduced noise level. Cindy, an exemplary nurse, confirmed this when she stated,

> In the end, their cognition and ability to perceive things around them is limited, or they may become hypersensitive to the softest sound. All they need is the sense that someone is there, so just being there and touching them is the best nursing care you can give.

Often, dying patients seem appreciative of silence. Silence gives patients time to evaluate what is happening, and it allows them to focus without disruption. An important part of preparing to die is life review — a reflection, an evaluation of one's life. This may be accomplished best in an environment that is quiet and free of distractions.

## When the news is bad

Throughout the course of their disease, cancer patients may receive news that is distressing. Diagnostic test results showing that the tumour has returned or reports that the treatment has not been effective can be emotionally devastating. In these instances, the nurses I studied most often chose silence as the most adequate nursing intervention.

While commenting about such situations, Jane advised, "They wouldn't understand your words, but they do understand your silence." This view was echoed by Moria, who said, "When something is too overwhelming, silence and touch are the only things that make sense." Marie commented, "When my patients get really bad news — something that just shatters them — I just sit with them and hold them. Anything that I can think to say at a time like that won't make it better. It's just too bad to be made better."

———

**SILENT SUPPORT**
Your words are lost
in a sea of confusion and pain.
They are not lifeboats for me,
they are like icebergs jamming me, ramming me,
pushing me under again, and again,
until I can't breathe.

Stop! Please stop.
Just stay with me and share my pain.

———

## When patients are psychologically or cognitively impaired

Frequently, patients with cancer have cognitive or psychological barriers that inhibit verbal communication. One field note reads,

> Cindy has to be so skilled at alternative forms of communication. Today, none of her three patients could communicate through speech. One is deaf, one only speaks Croatian, and one is heavily sedated and cognitively impaired by medication. Silent exchanges combined with touch were her only means of communicating important and complex messages to each of them.

Patients who are cognitively impaired or psychologically traumatized may take longer to respond to questions or statements from the nurse. Silence invites response and gives patients time to formulate an answer. The nurses I observed were sensitive to this. Julie told me, "With sick people you have to wait long enough to get a response.... If you are willing and able to wait, you just might find out something important, but first you have to be comfortable with silence." This was supported by Jane who commented, "I use silence. It gives patients psychological space to think — to change their minds."

For patients in denial, silence is very important. This is a story of a moment I observed, taken from my field notes.

> Sitting and staring at the TV was an attractive woman, probably about 30 years old, although it was hard for me to tell because she had lost all of her hair. When we entered her room, her gaze remained fixed on Oprah. The nurse walked up to her and sat down next to her. Without forcing eye contact, the nurse said, "Leigh-Ann, would you like to talk?" As the nurse sat waiting for a response, Leigh-Ann turned to her and in an angry outburst said, "There must be some mistake — it can't be me. This isn't happening. You must have the wrong person." Quickly the anger gave way to waves of sobs as the patient collapsed back into her chair. The nurse said nothing. In staying close and silent, she neither reinforced the denial nor impinged on the patient's need for it.

Blondis and Jackson explain how silence can be used to respond to a patient in denial. They recommend that, "you let your silence say, 'I am here, I will help you in any way I can. You are not alone.'"[28]

## When words are unnecessary

The nurses all described incidents in their practice where words were unnecessary. At times like these, they knew what their patients were thinking, or what they needed from them, without being told verbally. This story, written by Marie, is an example of one of these situations.

> Mimi was an exotic-looking Egyptian lady in her mid-twenties. A mother of three, she was a mere imprint

of her former self. Mimi was suffering from the "silent killer," ovarian cancer. A bowel obstruction prevented her from eating and she was being kept alive with intravenous nutrition. No further treatments aimed at curing her disease were planned.

Her youngest child was a year old. The room was dim, as the curtains were drawn. Her children were playing in the room away in a corner. I sat on her bed as she had called and asked me to come to her. The family members brought the baby to her. Mimi turned and looked at me. "Please take her," she said, pushing the baby towards me.

At first I was puzzled by her request, but soon I knew what was happening. I eagerly took the child and held her close to me. Mimi had begun to draw away from those she loved most. She would soon begin her new journey — the end was near. Yet she wanted to see that her loved ones would still be cared for after she was gone. My accepting her baby reassured her of this in a symbolic way.

I felt very special that she called me and asked me to hold her baby. I will always remember her. I didn't talk to her about that request. I knew what was happening, if only subconsciously. Silence was all that was needed. It gave her permission to separate, for now she was journeying alone.

—

**SILENCE IS FOREVER**
Words are for now;
silence is for eternity.

—

## When there are no right words

Sometimes no words are the right words. When this happened to Marie, she relied on silence.

Code one, one, one. My patient. My room. It was 0200 hours and staffing was minimal. My heart was pounding, adrenaline pumping. It was my patient who had arrested.

Fortunately, the cardiac response was strong and the arrest was primarily respiratory. He was in stable condition within 45 minutes of the beginning of CPR. I would give him one-to-one nursing care for the remainder of the night.

The next day I went to see him, as I felt I should share with him some of my thoughts during the code. I told him that I was very frightened that we might have lost him and that I was glad that he responded so well. He revealed that he was very much aware of our presence during the code. He remembered every detail of the experience. Then he pulled out a very carefully folded letter he had written his adult son. It contained instructions that he should not be resuscitated should this happen again. Tears dripped slowly down his cheeks as he read it to me. I listened intently for this was a very precious "sharing" gift to me. When he finished, we enjoyed a few moments of quiet togetherness. No verbal response was needed.

—

**UNSPOKEN WORDS**
The most powerful words
in the human language
may be those that are never said.

—

## THE GIFTS OF SILENCE

When a nurse is able to use silence effectively, patients benefit in several ways. These ways I called the gifts of silence: the gift of being present and the gift of listening with openness.

*Being present*
Silence allows the nurse to be more fully present in the encounter. This is a gift to the patient, but it is often equally positive for the nurse.

—

**THE GIFTS OF SILENCE**
With my silence I give you everything,
permission to cry,
to laugh,
to be silent too.

—

What does it mean to be present — to really be there for the patient? The literature promotes "presencing," or "being with" as one means by which nurses can assure patients they care about them. Bottorff states, "There is something in the 'being with' that reveals the nurse's feeling with the other, regard for the other as a person, and desire for the other's well-being."[29] Clayton, Murray, Horner, and Grene claim that presencing is a part of establishing a connection between nurse and patient.[30] To Watson, being present is an expression of the nurse's participation in the patient's experience.[31] Watson states that, "Human presence may in some ways directly and or indirectly

58

restore the human-centered subjectivity and dignity of both the care provider and care receiver."[32]

Presencing is more than just being physically present. Marcel, in a classic article, distinguishes between physical presence and being truly present.

> There are some people who reveal themselves as "present," that is to say at our disposal, when we are in pain or need to confide in someone, while there are other people who do not give this feeling, however great is their good will…. The most attentive and the most conscientious listener may give me the impression of not being present; he gives me nothing, he cannot make room for me in himself…. The truth is that there is a way of listening which is a way of giving, and another way of listening which is a way of refusing…. Presence is something which reveals itself immediately and unmistakably in a look, a smile…or a handshake.[33]

For Marcel, being present is communicated in part through silent measures: listening, looking, smiling, and touching.[34] As Green-Hernandez states, "Being there does not need to be verbally stated in order to be felt."[35] It is more than sitting or standing beside someone, or saying "I'm here for you." It involves an overlapping of selves, or as Watson describes it, it is a "human-to-human connectedness" where each is touched by the "human centre" of the other.[36] The nurses I interviewed talked about being there for their patients. Jane commented,

> The best way you can let your patients know you are there for them is by giving them silence. Staying with them through the silence tells them that you have time for them, that they are important to you — more

important than anything else at that moment. If it's quiet, and there are no more questions and no more answers required and you still stay with them, it tells them a lot. In our culture, a lull in the conversation is a chance to leave — to physically remove yourself. If that break comes and the patient finds you still there, they know you really want to be with them.

Marie simply said, "You can really be present when you are silent."

Being present with a patient is a choice made by the nurse. One must engage in self-discipline to gain skill in quieting and focusing one's self in order to be truly present for others. While the nurse may be concerned with fleeting time and tasks to be accomplished, the patient is focused on the moment. To be effective, the nurse needs to attend to what is important to the patients — their here and now experience.

What does being there do for the patient? It seems that it makes patients feel emotionally and physically safe. The following field note demonstrates this.

Her patient tonight can't talk. Each breath is a struggle. He is so afraid that the next breath just won't be there. In his eyes I see an unmistakable look of panic. A laryngeal cancer and tracheostomy have taken his vocal cords and a tonsillar tumour has impaired his hearing. How can she let him know that she is there, that she cares? She doesn't say a word. As she strokes his hair, her eyes tell him what he so desperately wants to hear: that she is with him, that she will stay, that she will watch over him. Gradually, silently, he drifts off to sleep.

Bottorff agrees with this view. She writes,

When a nurse is with us, in the sense of being present, we feel the security of her protective gaze, we feel valued as a person, the focus of her attention.... We sense the nurse is close enough to feel with us, sharing the loss that accompanies the dis-ease we are experiencing in a sensitive, intimate way.... She understands. When a nurse is truly present, seeing and feeling all these things, we sense a kind of hopefulness.... For a moment, we are not alone.[37]

A story written by Julie illustrates the power of silent presence.

My first encounter with Paul was on the phone. He had heard about palliative care but wanted to clarify a few things. I could hear young children playing happily in the background. I explained about symptom management, admission criteria, etc. I thought perhaps he had an ill parent. Who knows, maybe he was a reporter, a philanthropist, or maybe he wanted to volunteer? His questions were well prepared and specific. The closest I could get to asking, "Why do you want to know this anyway?" without feeling I had intruded, was saying, "We are here to help. Please feel free to call back if we can be of any further assistance."

Some weeks later a Paul was admitted to room 6. The door was always shut; his wife and his two children visited daily. He was waiting to die. He withdrew from everyone.

I could almost guarantee that, when I was on, he would be part of my assignment, as the other nurses find this kind of patient frustrating. It seems no matter what you give, nothing comes back. Finally, one day in sheer desperation, I heard myself saying, "Paul, this is Julie, your nurse. Yes, I'm your nurse again today. And I know this isn't fair, but you're just going to have to put up with me. You see, I am your nurse and you deserve just as much time as any of my other patients." As the scenario evolved, I spent time with him. Sometimes I would read to him — mostly, we would just be together.

In one way, he was still waiting for a miracle. One day we did discuss the whole thing of miracles. Yes, there was a miracle there; it wasn't the one he had hoped for, but it was there nevertheless. We celebrated his daughter's fourth and son's first birthdays on the unit. It was clear as the days passed that this little boy was his Dad's miracle. The spitting physical image of his Dad, he learned to walk in our long hallway. Both kids and Dad would take over our Jacuzzi tub with mountains and mountains of bubbles (Yes, they do plug the jets and you have to call maintenance to fix it!). You see, that little boy was conceived after Paul's diagnosis and was born with the astrological sign of Cancer. The odds said that Paul should have never seen his child born, never mind walk, say "Daddy," or demonstrate his Dad's incredible shyness.

Paul continued to be "my patient." The door was still closed most of the time and we still spent a lot of our time together without exchanging many words. But one day I will never forget as long as I have the privilege of living. I opened his door — not really knowing what I was going to encounter that day — to see him lying there with a single yellow rose in his hand and a card that said, "For Julie." We didn't say anything; we just hugged. I came out of that room and totally lost it. I don't usually hesitate to share tears with my patients, but for some reason, that day I really lost it. The sheer intensity of that moment, even as I write it down, still makes me cry.

—

**BREAKING THROUGH**

Words, words, words,

jackhammers pounding

against my protective wall of isolation.

They do not crack it.

Gentle, silent presence

passes through the wall,

and dismantles it,

without even leaving a mess.

—

## Listening with openness

Silence is important for listening and for hearing the message. You must be silent if you wish to listen to another — to listen with openness. Listening with openness involves silencing not only your mouth, but also your mind. Only if you are silent in these ways, can you receive and give the gift of listening with openness.

An exemplary nurse named Maureen said, "Good listening is an essential ingredient for providing nursing care of good quality." She went on to say, "Listening — listening is the biggest part of nursing. You need to be an active listener. The best nurses are the best listeners." Maureen then recalled a specific incident when, she believes, that really listening was all a patient needed from her.

Dani was a 32 year old woman who should have had the rest of her life ahead of her. She was married and had two young children — one four and one six months old. During her most recent pregnancy, she had noticed a change in a mole above her right eye. The surgical removal of the mole had been unsuccessful and the wide-spread metastases were diagnosed quickly after that. She developed a cord compression which didn't respond to radiation therapy, so she could no longer walk.

This particular incident occurred during her final admission. I was working nights and I had just finished my 0300 hour round. I entered Dani's room to find her wide awake staring out the window. I walked up to her and asked if she was having trouble sleeping. She said that she had been lying awake thinking about life and what she had accomplished. I asked her if she would like me to stay and sit with her awhile. She accepted, telling me how frightening nights could be. I put down her side rail and pulled up a nearby chair. I laid my hand on top of hers, and for an hour, I sat and listened to her. She told me how she had met her husband, about her university years, her brief career, her adventure in Europe, and finally about her two children. Her biggest regret was that she wouldn't be able to see them grow up. After she shared this with me, she seemed to relax. I started gently stroking her forehead, and she finally slept.

A common way we communicate understanding is by listening — not passively but actively, letting the person know they are being attended to, heard, and understood. Nurses have to be able to let their patients know that both the factual and the emotional content of what was communicated have been heard. This kind of active listening seeks the other's feelings. Succinctly stated, effective listeners are people who use silence with as much eagerness as they use talk.

—

**LISTENING WITH OPENNESS**
As I listen to you speak,
my ears catch the sound,
but my heart absorbs the message,
and I allow myself to be changed by your words.

In this way,
listening is a gift to you,
but it is equally a gift to me.

—

One way to listen effectively is by asking questions that encourage the patient to continue or to elaborate and then remaining quiet while he or she answers fully. The silence indicates compassion, acceptance, and support, as well as a willingness to be part of the patient's experience.

O'Banion and O'Connell provide a sensitive account of listening with openness:

All of me that I am in touch with and can command is directed toward you, what you are saying. All the facets of my being that feel are ready to receive your feelings. I begin to feel the struggle of your wanting to share with me; not being me, not trusting me, not knowing if I understand what it is you want to share. I feel your struggle and offer support. I want to understand. I know this is not easy for you. I lean toward you, I am ready to hear and feel, I am to be trusted. You share more, I do not retreat. I seem to want to understand. I seem to know what you are feeling. The pain grows strong and the tears relieve the pressure inside. I do not run away, I move closer, I touch a tear and say, "What do these mean?" Your pain touches the feeling of my pain and I respond with like pain. We share tears. I care for you.[38]

—

**THE DIFFERENCE**

When I hear—I hear.

When I listen—I feel.

I make room in myself for you.

—

### FORMS OF SILENCE

In observing the nurses, it was possible to identify several different forms of silence. Specifically, non-verbal messages framed in silence, silent messages encoded in words, and silent messages encoded in actions.

*Non-verbal messages framed in silence*

Non-verbal communication is a "two-way mime performed on the stage of the unconscious, conveying messages that are only partially transmitted verbally."[39] Non-verbal behaviour is a code that is impossible to fully describe, yet it can be understood by all.

Roberts and Bucksey suggest that non-verbal behaviour "includes all behaviors that convey messages without the use of verbal language."[40] Further, they note that attempts have been made to quantify the relative importance of verbal and non-verbal behaviours, with estimates of the non-verbal component ranging from 55 percent to 97 percent of the message. Despite the variations in these values, non-verbal aspects of communication are consistently thought to be more influential than verbal behaviours.[41]

Non-verbal behaviours can include gestures and movements, facial expressions, proximity, touch, self-touching, gaze, posture, gait, dress, accessories, and emblems. Researchers specify that certain non-verbal responses such as close proximity, prolonged eye contact, touch, and a calm, soothing voice can reassure the patient.[42]

During my time in the nursing unit, I observed that non-verbal gestures may be accompanied by words, the real message that is being communicated non-verbally is almost always framed in silence. The nurses seemed aware of this phenomenon and trusted the silent non-verbal messages over their patients' verbal responses.

Julie, the nurse in the case below, was sensitive to the non-verbal message being sent by the patient's mother. Although the message was subtle and could easily have been misinterpreted or ignored, Julie recognized a significant moment and captured the opportunity to help this woman.

The mom of an 18 year old girl with a brain tumour was standing outside her daughter's room, staring at the coffee maker, fumbling with her cup, and apparently about to pour herself one. Julie walked up to her and said, "You need a hug." She gave the mom an extended bear hug and, without further words, guided her to a private corner of the unit where they sat and talked.

The patient had just told her mom that when she died she would go to heaven and be a star shining down on everyone. This image had been too much for the mom to bear. After Julie talked to her, she was able to go back into the room and be with her daughter.

When I asked Julie about this encounter, she said, "Didn't you see the look in her eyes, and the way she was standing. She didn't want any coffee, she just couldn't bring herself to go back in the room. I could just tell she was ready to break." Julie had detected the non-verbal message framed in this family member's silence.

## Silent messages encoded in words

There were times during my observations when I saw the nurses seek, find, and decode silent messages, requests, and pleas from the in patients that were encoded in words that, on the surface, carried a completely different meaning. The delivery of high quality care depends on understanding patients' needs — many of which are expressed indirectly.

On one occasion, a patient rang her bell and, as Julie and I entered the room, the distressed woman said, "The baby won't settle and needs a little pat. Bring the baby here and I will give him a rub." As I looked around the room for a non-existent baby, the nurse, after pausing for a moment, turned the patient onto her side and gave her a back rub. Leaving a very content patient, Julie said to me, "I understood what she meant. She just needed a little attention herself." This same patient had been labeled as "confused" by some other staff members.

Sharp, accurate perception is a necessary ingredient of meaningful patient care. An exceptional nurse is discerning, knows the patients well, and is able to anticipate their needs by reading the silent messages in their words. For example, Julie told me,

What the patients say isn't always what they mean. Yesterday, I offered a patient a back rub. She said, "No, I'm okay." I just knew that she didn't want to say no. She really would have liked to say yes, but she didn't want to bother me or take any of my time. So I said, "Of course you are okay, but how about a treat." A big smile came across her face and I gave her the rub. We both felt good about it.

—

**HOLOGRAM OF LIFE**

Hidden in our everyday conversations,
are the things we would like to say
if we only had the courage.

——

To fulfill nursing responsibilities, many messages need to be communicated between nurse and patient. In an environment that is frequently emotionally laden, some of the messages that should be communicated are difficult to say. As a result, the encoding of messages in safe words occurs. This is an indirect way of saying what needs to be said. It can happen in conversations initiated by either the nurse or the patient. For example, Cindy called the son of a patient whose condition had deteriorated and said, "Your Dad's not able to be up at all today. He can't recognize any of us, and his breathing is poor." Translated this means, "Your Dad's probably dying. Please come quickly." I asked Cindy about this conversation and she explained it this way.

> In a situation like this, I usually try the gentle approach at first. If it doesn't work — if they just don't get it — I become as direct as I need to be to get my patient's needs met. I think the more subtle angle is good because it gives the person you are talking to a chance to come to the sad realization on their own. It's not forced on them. It's not so harsh, it's just more human somehow. But it is still honest, not just as directly honest.

Jane had this story about a patient's encoded message for her.

> It had been a very long day. I had six patients, all requiring complete care, so I was really tired. Mrs. Marshall was particularly time-consuming. She had cancer of the cervix that had spread throughout her abdomen. The draining fistulas around her groin area necessitated frequent dressing and linen changes. It was close to the end of my shift, and as I changed her bed and tucked her in, I managed a quick "bye" and hurried out of the room, anxious to go home. She called after me, "Thank you,

Jane. Take care of yourself." I replied, "okay, I will," and rushed down the hallway.

After I'd taken about 20 steps, I stopped. Something was wrong. It wasn't what she had said— it was how she said it. Mrs. Marshall was trying to tell me something. I went back to her side, took her hand and said, "You're saying goodbye, aren't you." She said that she knew her death was near and that she wouldn't see me again, but she wanted me to know how much my care had meant to her. I thanked her, too, for all that she had taught me about life and death. Then we said a proper goodbye.

The next morning when I went to her room it was empty. I would have been so sad if I hadn't heard her message.

———

### HIDE-AND-SEEK
Like children in the garden,
we play hide-and-seek with our words.
I hide, you seek.
You seek, I hide.
Back and forth we go.

Why do we play this game?
We really have no choice.
We need a cushion, a cloud around our words.
It keeps them from bumping into our emotions,
and breaking them to bits.

———

*Silent messages encoded in actions*

Cindy recounted situations in which she believed her actions transmitted powerful messages to her patients and the family members. In Cindy's estimation, silent messages can be encoded in nursing actions that communicate meaning more adequately than words can:

> Sometimes what the nurse does and how she does it communicates so much to the patient and family. When a patient is close to death for example, the family focuses on the small physical things like uncut toenails, uncombed hair, or wax in the ears. I make sure these things are all taken care of. It doesn't do much for the patient, but it reassures the family that all that can be done is being done and that I care about the patient.

In our conversations the nurses often referred to the importance of how they perform their work. They talked about being confident in their actions, meeting the patient's needs quickly, keeping the work environment neat, and keeping "inappropriate" staff behaviour out of the sight of patients. The major reason for this concern about how the care is delivered is summed up in Lana's comment:

> The patients and their families are always watching us. They determine how good we are by how we do things. How you do your work tells them a lot. They don't know if you are doing a procedure correctly or not, but they do know if you are working confidently. We want them to have confidence in us. We have to show them by how we meet their needs that they can trust us — that they matter to us.

Another exemplary nurse, Peter, said, "Doing the little things like folding their pajamas and putting them away in the morning, remembering to warm up their milk if they like it that way, bringing them two different flavors of jam to choose from — it might seem trivial, but it is critical."

This field note describes an example of Peter and his colleague being mindful of the small details in their care and the message this communicates.

> The patient is a very elderly Oriental lady. She is unable to speak or understand English. Today she is dying. They tend to her often, making sure she is comfortable. They select the prettiest nightgown from the hospital collection, a blue flowered one that complements her complexion. They choose one with long sleeves (because she is always cold). Every time they turn her, her hair is combed, her mouth and eyes are moistened. She is too weak to drink from a straw, so a few droplets of water are gently placed on her tongue. All of these actions are done with such gentleness. Their hands don't make a sound as they move from task to task.

During a conversation, Marie commented:

> I try to make my patients feel like they are the most important people in the world to me for the moments that I am with them. That has been my goal. It's the little things that make patients feel important — like the way you enter a room is important. I consciously slow down my pace as I go through their doorway. I attend to their needs in short order, not waiting to be reminded. If I can I anticipate their wants, like an extra pillow or a glass of juice, it makes a big difference to them. What I do and how I do it tells them so much.

Julie talked about the importance of another silent action:

> I try to always keep promises. If I say I'll be by to make
> their bed at 1000 hours, then I'm there at 1000 hours,
> not five minutes after. If I get busy, I stop by and tell
> them I will be delayed.... It tells them that they are
> important to me.

In all of these examples, the nurses are transmitting silent messages to
the patients, messages that are encoded in their actions. The nurse's
actions are observable by the patients, whose interpretation of their
actions may affect the nurse-patient relationship in many ways.

Because nursing work involves two-way communication, patients
also transmit silent messages in their actions. Cindy told me this
story about an elderly Russian gentleman:

> He couldn't speak a word of English. I had just finished
> making him a cup of tea because he loved tea with break-
> fast, and the kitchen staff always sent him coffee. When
> I brought him his cup, he didn't say anything — he just
> reached right up and kissed me.

—

**THE KISS**

When you meet my needs
you tell me that you care for me.
That even though I'm old and sick
I still have value,
I still have worth.
I kiss you.
It's the only way I have to say
I treasure what you do for me.
You keep me whole.

—

Cindy's example, like many of the others in this chapter, illustrates the two-way nature of silent communication. Silence is used by both the patients and the nurses during their encounters. In this way, it is a dialogue of silence.

### REFLECTIONS ON THE DIALOGUE OF SILENCE

Each of the qualities of silence suggested at the opening of this chapter — purity, precision, and perfection — are discussed in the following reflective summary.

### The purity of silence

Words are often not what they seem and are sometimes used to camouflage what is actually felt. From the observations and interviews, as well as my past experience, it appears that silence provides the purest form of communication.

Wordless messages are not likely to be interpreted in any way by the sender before they are sent. When we use words to communicate, we are in a sense analyzing our own thoughts before sending them. To put a feeling into words, we usually first think of what we are trying to say and then of how it can be phrased. We may decide to couch, or limit, the expression of our true emotions, needs, or thoughts by the words we choose. However, when we send a message in silence, it is uncontaminated by words that are open to misinterpretation by the receiver, or limitation by the sender.

Silence does not have to be used alone. It is often combined with other non-verbal and verbal forms of communication. Doing so does not diminish its purity and may sometimes increase its effectiveness, such as when silence is combined with appropriate touch. At other times silence is best left unadulterated and untreated, just whole and real.

## Silence is precise

If we were to depend on words alone to communicate our needs, fears, hopes, and feelings, not only would our communication be susceptible to inaccuracies, it would be slow. Words are often not efficient; they may be imprecise and awkward. It frequently takes many words to convey a single emotion, and then, when one's feelings are put into words, they can be misinterpreted.

Alternatively, a silent moment can convey a myriad of emotions — precisely, quickly, and accurately. Jane, in analyzing a narrative she had written, said, "Silence is more filled with communication than words can ever be."

Not only are words often inadequate and lacking in precision, they can be destructive to the nurse-patient relationship. Phrases like, "It will be okay," "I know how you feel," and "Don't worry," are not only ineffective, they can convey a message that is the antithesis of what the words are meant to say. When we were discussing this notion, Moria commented,

When I'm tempted to say something like, "You'll be fine," an alarm goes off in my head and I just shut up. Saying, "You'll be fine," is like saying, "I really don't care about you or your situation. I'm uncomfortable with you sharing your feelings with me. I don't know how to answer you. Please stop talking." It doesn't do the patient any good at all. You are better off saying nothing.

—

**SHARPENED WORDS**
Words between us are few.
But the words we do share,
these words are like arrows,
sharpened by the silence.

—

75

Blondis and Jackson provide a succinct summary of how a nurse's actions without words can communicate with great precision.

> It does not take a lot of words to tell patients you really care. You tell them best by going directly to them as you enter the room, staying close to them, physically touching them, and asking them with your eyes what their needs are.[43]

## Silence is perfect

Silence is a vessel for carrying messages. It is limitless in capacity, and nearly always free of defects. In silent messages, there is little of the message lost. The silent meaning goes by a direct route, from the mind of the sender to the mind of the receiver. It is not filtered first through a mesh of imprecise words. Although non-verbal gestures can be deliberately performed and are open to misinterpretation, silence is largely exempt from these frailties. Silence takes non-verbal communication to a higher level of interpersonal exchange.

Silence is especially effective for transmitting feelings and emotions, things that we do not have words for. Compassion, acceptance, and support are communicated best by silence. In an emotionally laden environment, these communications are frequently necessary, and often the words we have available are too limited to communicate such subtle and intense meanings and messages.

When silence is used constructively, the nurses can have stronger ties with their patients. Physiologically, psychologically, and spiritually there are times when patients need silence. If the nurses can recognize these times, they can be very effective caregivers. Silence gives patients, their families, and the nurses what they are often lacking in the very public environment of a hospital: privacy and psychological space.

In silent moments, the spirits of both the patient and the nurse can be nurtured. Perhaps perfect silence can be the ultimate encounter between nurse and patient — as Watson suggests, an opportunity for the restoration of the human dignity of both the care-provider and the care-receiver.[44]

Taylor writes, "Silence is not void, but productive...silence rings."[45] Caputo, in like vein, asserts that to "hear what is spoken in silence, all voices and sounds must be put away and a pure stillness must be there, a still silence."[46]

Such silence is crisp, clear, and pristine. Creating a space where stillness can be found provides an atmosphere where patients are listened to and understood, where messages are sent and received unblemished by the static of the airways. For this to happen, the nurse must have the self-discipline, combined with awareness of self and situation, to remain appropriately silent.

Jane shared this story of her discovery of the impeccability of silence.

> It was such a cold February day. My patient had just died. The family hadn't made it in time. I felt so sorry that I did not call them sooner. As they arrived on the elevator, I greeted them without words and took them to the bedside. We stood huddled together in silence. I remember thinking at the time, "My God, it's so quiet. This is so good. This is just what we need." In the privacy of our own thoughts, we were each able to come to a realization of the meaning of the loss for each of us.

—

**PERFECT SILENCE**
Someday,
after we understand
the genetic code of all life forms,
the components of all universes,
the intricacies of all human interactions,
we will understand and use silence.

Then,
for the second time
in the history of the human race,
we will have learned to fly.

—

# *chapter four*

## MUTUAL TOUCH

Of my three main themes of exceptional nursing care, the second is what I call "mutual touch." This chapter develops the theme of mutual touch using my field notes, the words of the exceptionally competent nurses I studied, and again, poems combined with narrative comments.

I define what mutual touch means to me, and discuss the importance of touch in health care to provide some context for my descriptions of eight types of touch that I observed exemplary nurses using: procedural, non-physical, talking, trigger, social, diagnostic, comforting, and the final touch.

I examine the nature of 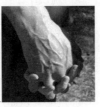 touch and explore what touch is, how it fits in our society, how culture affects touch, the qualities of touch, touch as a language, and how touch can be used with other mediums of communica- tion. Throughout the chapter, I refer to the nursing literature on the use of touch in effec- tive health care.

## MUTUAL TOUCH DEFINED

Touch by its nature is reciprocal; it affects both the person initiating the touch and the person being touched. It is impossible to touch someone without also being touched yourself; therefore, touch is a shared activity. As this opening poem suggests, perhaps both the nurse and the patient are affected when a touch occurs.

—

**THE HUG**

Arms entwined.

Warmth exchanged.

Heart beats felt.

Concern sensed.

Care given.

Care given.

—

Early in my observations of exceptionally competent nurses, it became evident that touch was important in the care given. These care providers used every opportunity to touch their patients in a spectrum of ways to accomplish a variety of purposes. Touch seems to be one way they make a connection. One field note reads,

> She often sits on the bed next to her patients, or she stands very close to their chairs. This physical closeness seems to create an air of familiarity. It makes their relationship close very quickly. With these nurses and their patients, there is a sense of urgency.... They seem to be saying, "We might not have too long; let's cut through the formalities; let's not play games; let's invite each other in right away."

After another day in the unit, I recorded this observation on the use of touch.

It was by touching, by holding her hand, laying a cold cloth on her forehead, and rubbing her sore back, that the nurse communicated that she cared. All that she did with touch said how much she wanted to help.

## THE IMPORTANCE OF TOUCH IN HEALTH CARE

The debate between the importance of touch versus technology in nursing was happening as early as 1982 when Naisbitt wrote, "We must learn to balance the material wonders of technology with the spiritual demands of our human nature" because "when high tech and high touch are out of balance, dissonance results."[47] In agreement with this point of view Tough adds, "Beyond technology nurses have much to offer patients, they can offer themselves as well as their hands."[48]

Upon entering a hospital, people encounter an unfamiliar, aseptic environment. Uniformed caregivers move swiftly about the maze of corridors. Steel-wheeled chairs and stretchers clatter, and machines flash and beep. The alien odour of antiseptic solution drenches the air. Hospitalization is a frightening, disorienting, depersonalizing experience.

In such an environment, Watson points out, "The caregiver provides a human presence that touches another's mind or spirit."[49] Human touch becomes imperative. It restores the human element, telling patients in a concrete way that there are caring people here. Touch can reach past the bureaucratic-technological system and scientific treatment, allowing the patient to reach out of the solitude of suffering.

While in hospital, a patient's psychological well-being is threatened. There is depersonalization and sensory deprivation. The effect is anxiety provoking. Ryan adds that anxiety is among the most common and strongest responses to hospitalization.[50] This point is also made by Sims who explains that anxiety associated with the stress of hospitalization must be countered by intervention involving caring, touch, and human contact.[51]

One branch of the caregiving community which has recognized the importance of touch is nursing. Montagu attributes the use of touch by nurses to two conditions. First, the majority of nurses are women, and second, nursing tasks often require that nurses are in close physical proximity to their patients. He concludes that nurses have been in a far better position to appreciate the importance of touching in the care of the patient, and therefore it has become a natural part of nursing.[52] In agreement with Montagu, Bottorff contends that touch is universal and basic to the nurse-patient relationship.[53]

One of my field notes describes the liberal use of touch by an exceptional nurse.

> The use of touch is very evident. On entering the room of almost every patient, the nurse takes the patient's hand, or places a hand on their shoulder. The nurse almost always goes to the patient's face, instead of addressing a patient from the foot of the bed or the doorway. Standing close, making physical contact, and talking directly to their patient is the most common position these nurses take.

Marie said, "Nursing is wonderful because you get to touch the patient." Jane states, "Touch is used by nurses in different ways than it is used by other caregivers. Doctors touch the patients because they have to. We touch the patients because we choose to."

The nature of the nurse-patient relationship is such that touching is both inescapable and acceptable. Touch is the most personal of our senses because it brings two human beings into physical contact. To carry out nursing procedures, the nurse must move into the patient's personal space. Barraja-Rohan explains that everyone has this personal space — an invisible area that surrounds their body. This space, the author claims, is dynamic and varies from person to person.[54] Only by decreasing the physical distance and crossing into this area are the touching behaviours such as holding, hugging, grasping, and stroking possible. The physical space of both the patient and the nurse overlap when one touches the other.

Although it is understood that nurses move into the patient's physical space to provide care, the nurse must also be willing to accommodate the patients in their own spaces. For it to be a meaningful touch in which messages are communicated and received, there is usually unspoken agreement that both are willing for this encounter to occur.

Nurses have implicit permission to touch patients because of their role. Benner emphasizes the unique role of nurses in that, "By their very position, nurses are asked different questions and looked to for different kinds of help than other professionals."[55] Julie expresses a similar view. She said, "Nursing invites you into places you would never go, across the barriers to people, holding their hands and being close." As Routasalo concludes, touch is an integral part of nurse-patient interaction in virtually all nursing situations.[56] The more the patient needs help in daily activities, the more the nurse will try to help by means of touching. After completing a review of the literature related to nursing and touch, Routasalo concludes that, in spite of its obvious importance, touch has received only marginal attention in nursing studies.[57]

The nurses' comments and stories reflected a belief in the importance of touch in nursing care. Jane states, "Touching is critical. Empathy, caring, love, and concern are all transferred through your eyes and hands." Lana emphatically proclaimed, "Touching — I think it is necessary. I think it is mandatory." After a particularly demanding day, Moria commented, "I like to leave a bit of myself behind for my patients. I do that with my touches.... I hope that the feeling of being safe and cared about that I communicate to them with my touch lingers on after I have gone. I believe that it does." Cindy confided, "I have had a really good day when I have made a connection with a patient — feeling comfortable sitting on their bed or giving them a hug, touching them in some way."

## THE NATURE OF TOUCH

In the following sections, various aspects of touch are addressed in an attempt to bring the reader to a greater understanding of the nature of touch. Specific mention is made of the use of touch in our society, the culture-specific influences on the use of touch, the qualities of touch, the language of touch, and the potential in combining touch with other mediums of communication.

### What is touch?

Touch is a powerful, sometimes disregarded, always complex channel of interpersonal communication. Chang describes touching as a therapeutic event, an avenue of connection and communication having physical, emotional, social, and spiritual significance with potential positive impacts on patients' well-being and comfort.[58] Watson contends that touch causes the dissolution of boundaries between two persons.[59] It is described by Langer-Albert and Short as a conductor of messages,[60] and by Montagu as capable of "soothing ruffled feelings, assuaging pain, relieving distress, giving reassurance, and making all the difference in the world."[61] Gadow called touch philanthropic, a gift from one who is whole to one who is not.[62]

Benner goes further, describing touch as a conveyer of "messages as well as physical stimulation and comfort."[63] She emphasizes that touch signifies an emotional involvement on the part of the nurse, a concern or caring for another. Watson agrees saying "Touch is concern made tangible…an expression of the nurse's participation in the patient's experience."[64]

We struggle with putting into words that which seemingly lies beyond words. Because of this sense of helplessness with the language, we turn to touch, the silent communication. Barraja-Rohan supports this assessment, adding that touch is always individualized and the interpersonal communications that happen through touch achieve a significance that verbal language cannot achieve.[65]

Referring to the shared nature of touch, Montagu writes, "Touch differs from all other senses in that it always involves the presence, at once and inseparable, of the body we touch and our body with which we touch it."[66] Touch is automatically reciprocal. A nurse cannot touch a patient without also being touched. In this way, the nurse and patient share the experience. Touch is a way to reassure another person that you are present in the fullest sense of the word.

The exemplary nurses, when discussing their touching behaviors, emphasized the importance of touch being genuine to be effective, to achieve this sense of being there for the patient. They said, "The touching has to develop in time. When I touch someone or embrace them, it has to be real for me, too." "It needs to be real. If it's phony, forget it." "It can't be forced. You have to be comfortable with it yourself first."

Although it obvious that many nursing interventions involve the use of hands and touch, the concept of touch is still not well developed in the literature.[67-69] It has been suggested that the subjectivity involved in touch and multiple variables of touch may be the reasons for the lack of research regarding physical touch.[70-72]

## Touch in society today

Although there is agreement that touch is an important interpersonal method of communication, fundamentally necessary for development and maintenance of health, Barraja-Rohan explains that it is increasingly being denied many people.[73] In Montagu's words, "Cuddling, caressing, embracing, stoking, the basic human touches, are withheld from the majority of people in our society."[74]

When a person is sick, disfigured, and deformed from cancer and cancer treatments, the withdrawal of human contact would seem even more likely. Withdrawal happens at a time when the benefits of touch are critically needed. Jane observed, "The elderly and dying especially hunger to be touched. Many of my patients — when I offer them my hand, they clasp it so tightly like it is a lifeline or some treasure they are guarding. Sometimes they even reach for me before I reach for them." Cindy said, "Touch seems especially important for the elderly patients…. Their hearing and vision are not good, and they are often starving for touch." Researchers support these observations, explaining that in older adults and the chronically ill especially, the need for tactile stimulation is a hunger which often remains unsatisfied.[75,76]

## Touch and culture

Montagu cautions that a wide range of class and cultural differences in attitudes and practices related to tactile behavior exists.[77] The nurses I studied were cognizant of these cultural variances and respected their patients' beliefs and preferences.

During a conversation, Marie remarked, "I am quite reserved about touch initially. I stand back at first and see what dance they want to dance. I think it's just good nursing to assess it. Not all the same approaches work for every patient, or every nurse."

Routasalo emphasizes that patients from varying backgrounds may differ in both the manner in which they express the need for touch and the manner in which they satisfy it, but the need is universal and is everywhere the same.[78] To be truly beneficial, it is apparent that tactile communication must be used appropriately, taking cultural mores into consideration.

## The qualities of touch

The qualities of touch can vary. To be effective in patient care situations, certain elements of touch are most desirable. For example, caring is transmitted through touching that is neither rushed nor rough in quality.

Bartenieff and Lewis detail three different qualities of touch: the fleeting light poke, the constrictive two-dimensional grip, and the three-dimensional enveloping hold.[79] They describe the three-dimensional touch as slightly bound in nature and explain that it communicates reassurance and support to the patient. In their opinion, this non-linear, total touch is the most effective in nurse-patient relationships; "A perfunctory peck on the cheek is no substitute for a warm embrace, nor is a conventional handshake capable of replacing a caressing hand."[80]

The nurses I interviewed also identified different qualities of their touches. Being mindful of the importance of individualizing their care, the nurses suggested that they were careful to use touches with which their patients felt comfortable. Marie commented,

> The last thing I want to do is scare one of my patients or their families members off because they feel smothered by my physical attention. I try to fit the approach to the patient. Sometimes it's hard to tell with people. If you just talk to them, they may seem reserved and not very demonstrative. But if you do take the risk and give them a little test hug, they usually cling on very tightly.

It is difficult to determine some qualities of a touch from a distance. As an observer, I could not determine the amount of pressure (whether hard or soft, light or heavy) and the temperature (whether warm or cold) of touches. However, it was possible to see that the touches used by the exceptionally competent nurses were gentle, not rough, and deliberate and slow rather than rushed. This observed moment provided an example:

> "What can I do to help you sleep better on your first night with us?" the nurse asks a newly admitted patient. The patient, a very frail cachexic man, is withdrawn and reserved. He says nothing.
>
> Not giving up, the nurse makes suggestions. "How about a back rub or a foot rub?" She watches the patient for a

clue, and when he smiles slightly at the mention of a foot rub, they set a mutually agreeable time for it to occur.

It is one of the most genuine messages of caring I can imagine. The lights are dimmed, the lotion warmed, her voice is soft and often silent. She stands at the foot of his bed so she can look at him as she does her work. Although her night is hectic, she takes her time, moving slowly and lovingly. When she is finished, she wraps his feet in warmed towels to prolong the physical and psychological effects after she is gone. The message that he is still an important and worthy person, and that she cares for him, is clearly communicated through her touch that some would say is not necessary. He wouldn't agree.

—

**YOU HAVE THE TOUCH**

The touch.

Soft,

gentle,

deliberate,

warm.

Comfort made tangible.

—

## The language of touch

In the literature, touch has been described as a language. Montagu suggests it is the language of the senses.[81] Tactile symbols create the language of touch, producing a channel of communication. Different qualities of touch, used in various combinations, are like the phrases of the language. Messages are communicated through this channel. The repetitive nature of touch is like the repetition of words in the language. Repetition in touch adds emphasis the same way that repetition in spoken language does.

88

—

**REPETITIVE TOUCH**

I move my hand over yours,

over and over and over.

I don't want to just say,

"I am here for you."

I want to say it very loudly.

—

The language of touch can communicate affection and warmth,[82] acceptance and support,[83] caring,[84] and it can reassure.[85] Like other languages, these exceptional nurses believe the language of touch can be learned. Many spoke of learning it through experience. Marie noted,

> In the beginning, I never touched my patients except to do care. It took me a long time to get comfortable with it; it took me a long time to learn to look past what I was seeing in the bed and see the real person lying there and to feel all right about touching them. Part of it was experience — life experience and nursing experience. Maybe part of it, too, is just being more comfortable with yourself and the situation.

## TOUCH COMBINED WITH OTHER MEDIUMS OF COMMUNICATION

Touch is seldom used in isolation, as the sole means of communicating with a patient. Regularly, as nurses touch their patients and their patients touch them, they also engage in other verbal or nonverbal interactions. Most commonly, silence and eye contact were combined with touch.

### Touch and silence

Touch and silence are often combined; although touch may be accompanied by words, it is frequently more meaningful without them. There are times when the best expressions of empathy and concern are in non-verbal touch. The following is an example of how touch and silence were combined to provide support for a family member.

> Her husband of many years has just died from his cancer. She has been out of the room making calls to relatives as the nurse tidies up the patient's room and prepares the body. The wife enters the room and, approaching the nurse, says, "How can I thank you?" and begins to cry. The nurse embraces her in a tight, enfolding hug. For a few minutes, the wife sobs softly into the nurse's shoulder. As she cries, the nurse continues the hug.
>
> When the crying stops, the nurse gently releases her and wipes her tears with a tissue that has been waiting in her pocket for just such a crisis. Maintaining contact with the wife by keeping her arm around her shoulder, the nurse walks the woman to the elevator. No words are ever spoken. No words are needed.

—

**MAGNIFIED TOUCH**

Silence,

a magnifying glass

for touch.

—

## Touch and eye contact

The emotional truth is often expressed non-verbally. Montagu suggests that non-verbal messages expressed through eye contact are very powerful. He adds, "The eyes have a language of their own."[86] When the languages of touch and eye contact are combined, messages that might otherwise be conveyed very awkwardly in words are exchanged instantly and emphatically.

As Montagu explains, "There is something about eye contact

90

that is almost palpable,"[87] and when it is combined with touch, there seems to be a synergistic effect resulting in a potent communication medium. Because of the intensity created in the combination, touch and eye contact were used together discriminately by the nurses being observed, with some caution and with respect. Usually these moments were short. They often occurred in emotionally charged situations where people either did not know what to say, or wanted to say more than words would seem to allow. This is an example of such a moment I witnessed:

> She had been a star, an entertainer, a celebrity. Now breast cancer had robbed her of her dignity and her wish to live. On two occasions she had tried without success to hasten her departure from this world. Moments ago, the nurse had discovered in her belongings enough medication to end her life. At the moment of this disclosure, their eyes met and stayed locked as the nurse walked to her and took her hand. For several seconds they maintained this stance, frozen together in time.

—

**ABSOLUTE CONNECTION**
Entranced in your eyes,
the messages come strongly and swiftly.
As you reach out and touch me,
you complete the circuit.
For a moment we are one,
understanding each other completely.

—

## TYPES OF TOUCH

It is difficult to label a particular touch as belonging to a single category, although certain touches seemed to fulfill specific purposes. A particular touch encounter, however, may achieve a variety of objectives and carry multiple messages. Each touch experience is unique and can be a very private experience between the participants. The stories of the nurses in the study provide insight into the experience from the nurse's perspective, and the observations capture only what could be seen. On occasion, I did ask the nurse to comment on a touch encounter I had observed, to provide additional insight.

In the following discussion, the examples of touches observed and recorded in discussion and narrative exchange have been grouped according to their apparent primary purpose. Going beyond the types of touches described in the literature, eight different types of touch were identified through analysis of the study data: procedural touch, non-physical touch, talking touch, trigger touch, social touch, diagnostic touch, comforting touch, and the final touch.

*Procedural touch : When a touch is more than a touch*
Patients are touched as part of many nursing procedures. However, how a nurse touches a patient during these procedures communicates a great deal about the nurse's feelings for that patient as a person. In this way, a procedural touch may be more than a touch for task-related purposes.

In Bottorff's study of the uses of touch by oncology nurses, the task-oriented or procedural touch was the one most frequently employed by the nurses she observed.[88] It is the touch that is part of the performance of nursing tasks, such as starting an intravenous line, administering medications, or changing a dressing. If nurses are accomplishing their technical duties, these touches are necessary.

The exemplary nurses I studied did use procedural touches. However, the procedures were done in such a manner that the touches took on certain qualities. These nurses made therapeutic use of the task-oriented touches, taking the opportunity to do their "work" and meet some of the patients' emotional needs simultaneously. For example, when they inspected a subcutaneous needle site, they touched the patient to fulfill this procedure, but they did so gently, without rushing to open the gown to access the location. Their actions communicated their concern and respect for the patient.

Often a procedural touch was accompanied by a secondary touch that was not required to complete the task. A squeeze of the hand, a stroke of the arm, or a caress of the face, said, "I care about you." In this way, an instrumental and expressive touch were combined.

As they performed interventions, these nurses were able to remain focused on the patients. By maintaining eye contact and talking to the patient when it was not critical that they be looking at the site of the intervention, they increased the patient's comfort with the situation and sometimes gathered important data. For example, they were able to assess how a patient was tolerating a procedure as it was being done, and then modified their approach if it was causing the patient physiological or psychological distress. If a procedure was potentially embarrassing or painful for the patient, the nurses were careful to maintain emotional contact by touching the patient throughout the process.

One specific procedural touch that was used liberally and effectively by most of the nurses I observed was the bath. Jane commented on the importance of bathing patients. She said, "Perhaps it is the symbolic nature of water as the source of life, maybe it is the comfort provided by warmth on sore joints, or it could be the stimulation from water pressure on the skin, but whatever the reasons, nurses love to bathe their patients."

Other nurses made comments about their use of bathing as an opportunity to communicate with their patients. They also talked about the tactile stimulations of the bath, the whirlpool jets, and the bubbles. Julie laughed and commented,

> We really do wash our patients a lot, probably more than
> we need to. Let's face it, they usually don't get really dirty.
> I think it is a form of therapy. When you combine the

stimulation of the water on the skin and the rubbing and scrubbing, it does more than just stimulate their circulation.... It makes them feel much better.

Moria also supported the importance of bathing patients saying, "I give every patient some kind of bath every day. It's a great time to talk to the patients.... There is something about that situation — all the barriers are removed with the clothes, and we really talk." Finally, Lana made this observation, "Giving someone a bath is such an intimate time. I can't think of any better way to get to know my patients."

The dressing change is another nursing procedure that involves touching. This account from my notes on an observed dressing change illustrates the combination of procedural touch with secondary touch.

The old dressing is gently removed. As she works, she watches the patient's eyes and face to see how he is tolerating the procedure. Carefully the wound is cleaned, but before applying the antiseptic, she warns the patient the solution may feel cold. The nurse accurately applies a new dressing. As she spreads the tape to hold the gauze in place, she rubs her hand on the skin around the wound site. She asks the patient if it feels all right and makes necessary minute adjustments. As she leaves the room, she give his hand a squeeze and winks at him. They exchange a smile.

In another field note, I recorded this observation of a nurse starting an intravenous line.

She enters the patient's room and explains the doctor has requested that an intravenous be started. In a careful and complete manner, she explains the procedure and what the patient can expect. Returning a few minutes later with the equipment, she applies the tourniquet over the patient's pajama sleeve so as not to pinch the skin beneath. Gently, she rubs the patient's skin to increase circulation so she can locate the vein. As she rubs, she looks at and talks to the patient. Before she inserts the needle, she warns the patient that there will be pain. She asks the patient how the needle feels, completes the procedure efficiently, and reassures the patient as she leaves by squeezing her shoulder. The nurse places the call bell within the patient's reach and asks the patient to call if she has any concerns.

These observations demonstrate how the exceptionally competent nurses approached two different nursing procedures. The dressing is complete and the intravenous is started, but in each situation the patient's feelings are respected while they are comforted and reassured through touch.

### Non-physical touch

The second type of touch observed was the non-physical touch. In exploring this area, I saw examples that supported Estabrook's claim that touch can be more than skin to skin contact.[89] Any modality that allows the human presence to be felt is, in a way, a form of touch. Music, art, literature, intellectual exchange, and non-contact physical closeness could all be viewed as variations of touch that might be called non-physical.

The exemplary nurses found ways to touch their patients non-physically. Peter, was especially skilled at what I called encircling. He would seldom lay a hand on the patient other than to perform procedural touches, but would often have his arm just behind the patient's back or around the patient's shoulders. Although no physical contact was made, I sensed that the feeling of support was present.

The following is an excerpt from a letter I wrote to Peter summarizing some of my observations of our time together.

> I was most affected by your gentleness of manner and by the tenderness of your touch. Your hands are so amazing. Even from a distance, I could sense an aura of warmth flowing from them. You have no need to physically touch your patients because you have the ability to encircle them with compassion and caring without direct contact. What power! Your patients are very fortunate to have you as their nurse.

My corresponding field note said, "He doesn't touch as much as he is physically close...and looks directly at the patients, staying at eye-contact level. He encircles them with his warmth without direct contact."

Montagu suggests eye contact is a variation of non-physical touch. He calls eye contact "touching at a distance."[90] In conversation, Julie echoed this view when she said, "To me, touching is critical. It communicates empathy, caring, affection, concern.... All of this is transferred through touches with your hands and touches with your eyes." Levine describes eye-contact touching as "looking through soft eyes."[91] Soft eyes, he claims, allow you to see with the heart. I believe this is often the way that the nurses I observed looked at their patients.

—

**SOFT EYES**
Your eyes throw light at me.
Some of it I store—my source of hope,
some of it I consume—my source of energy,
some of it I reflect—our source of unity.

—

## Talking touch

What are the messages embedded in touch? At certain times, when it seemed inappropriate or too difficult to use words, or the right words to communicate a feeling could not be found, touch was used. I have labeled this type of touch talking touch. Bartenieff and Lewis describe touch as "the authentic voice of feeling."[92] They conclude, "like music, [touch] often utters the things that cannot be spoken. Nothing need be said, for everything is understood."[93]

In some ways, talking touches share similarities with Bottorff's category of comforting touch.[94] Comforting touches, by Bottorff's definition, are given for the purpose of calming, soothing, quieting, reassuring, or encouraging patients. Although talking touches do in part meet these goals, they also are used to communicate a variety of additional messages. As the following examples illustrate, talking touches can be used to give patients specific messages or directions and are a vehicle for the nurses to share their feelings with patients and family members. The following field note describes the use of talking touch by one nurse.

As she cared for the patient and the grieving family, she never said, "I really care," but she said it many times non-verbally by her gentle touching of the patient. Her concern with keeping him comfortable in his final hours — hair combed, mouth and lips moist, her willingness to be the someone close by when the family faced the final moment — all told the family what they needed to hear.

Hagen found in her doctoral research that touch communicates the feeling of love.[95] Touches such as stroking, caressing, and cradling show involvement, concern, responsibility, tenderness, and awareness of the needs, sensibilities, and vulnerabilities of the other person.

In one of my field notes, I documented how Marie communicated a multitude of feelings to the patient and family members through talking touches.

> The patient is very ill — in fact, actively dying. As the wife and daughter pace anxiously in the hallway outside his room, the nurse approaches them and touches each on the arm as if to say, "I see how difficult this is for you." She leads them into the room and pulls a chair close to each side of the bed, encouraging them to sit with him and hold his hands. From time to time, the nurse gently places her hand on his pulse or touches his extremities, monitoring him closely but unobtrusively. The priest, summoned by the nurse at family's request, prays for the patient; as he does the wife looks questioningly at the nurse. She responds to the non-verbal question of "How much longer?" by placing her arm around the wife's shoulders. The patient dies peacefully. The nurse beckons the family to follow her down the hall to a quiet room where they can sit for a while. She stays with them, sitting close by and touching them often as they cry.

In talking with Marie later about this moment, she said, "Sometimes those little touches just let the patient or family member know that I am there for them. What I am meaning to say is I'm available to you in this time of need."

Some exemplary nurses indicated they use touch to communicate to patients that they are important to them. Jane commented, "If I think about why I do what I do…I always use a person's name, stand close, look at them, and touch them lightly on the hand or forearm as I speak. To me, this tells them that I am not too busy for them and that I do care."

Touch was used to talk to the patients when the news was too sad or difficult to be put into words. Julie remarked, "When the patient has just heard some really terrible report from the doctor, there is absolutely nothing to say that will match the intensity of the emotion." Lana agreed, "Bad news can only be met with touch. Putting it into words and talking about it right away make it too real. Nobody can bear it — not the patient or me. At times like that, I just hold them."

—

**NO MATCH**

Stumbling over my tongue,
words are a feeble match for the
relentless pounding of grief.

—

### Trigger touch

This story provides an example of a trigger touch — a touch that elicits the release of pent-up emotion in the person touched.

> Her husband was only 30, dying a slow painful death from stomach cancer. She was so strong — sitting by his bed all day, sleeping by his side at night, eating all of her meals next to him. The days stretched into weeks and still she stoically sat, asking the nurses and doctors for very little as she met most of her husband's physical and emotional needs. I wondered about her pain and I worried about her. I sought an opportunity to get inside, and finally one day it came.
>
> His supper tray was late, and she was pacing the halls awaiting its arrival. Her forehead was riveted with strain and anger. I approached her slowly, silently — and when we were close in physical distance, I touched her elbow and said, "It looks to me like you are sitting on the edge of tears. Can you share them?" In a great guttural cry, the weeks of frustration and anguish poured freely.

—

**JUST ONE TOUCH**
Just one spark,
can start the forest burning.
One rock removed,
begins the avalanche.

A single touch
can prompt a stampede of emotion,
the strength of which
could make any iron man shiver and shake
and beg for mercy.
But don't be afraid.
Unlike the fire and the avalanche
that bring destruction,
once the stampede of emotion has past,
genuine calm can prevail.

—

Moria observed, "Anger, sadness, or despair may come rushing out as a hand laid on a shoulder or a hug says, 'I'm here for you; I care about you; you can trust me with yourself.'" Watson supports this observation saying that touch may release a person from self-absorption or suffering.[96]

In conversation, Cindy told me that she watches for critical talking moments — times when a patient or family member who has been under stress "looks ready to let it go." She said, "Most times it's a little touch combined with a few words that give them permission not to hold it in any longer."

I observed Cindy using the approach she described. The wife of a man whose condition had been deteriorating daily was sitting outside her husband's room reading. Approaching the woman, Cindy knelt before her and, taking her hand, said, "You must be tired." With that small gesture, the words, worries, and tears that had been stored up for many days came out without hesitation.

In analyzing her approach, Cindy said, "It is a risk every time you do something like this. You might get rejected — verbally or non-verbally — but usually they really want to talk; they just need to be given the chance. You also have to be prepared to deal with whatever you uncover."

### Social touch

Bottorff identified a form of touch she called social touch.[97] By her definition, social touch is human physical contact that fosters social bonds, attachment, and permits individuals to maintain their emotional integrity. Montagu explains that, "cheek patting, hair patting, and clucking under the chin, in the Western world, are forms of behaviour indicating affection and social recognition."[98]

In my observations, many of the playful touches such as pretend punches, taps on the nose or cheek, or toes pulled gently were all touches of a social nature. Such physical contacts were made appropriately either during moments that were less emotionally intense or to diffuse a difficult situation.

Some social touches seemed to convey a sense of friendliness and playfulness between the two people involved. For example, I observed one nurse trying to get a response from a patient who, although he was physically quite well, had been lying in bed, staring at the ceiling and refusing to interact with anyone since his admission two days earlier. In my field notes I wrote,

> Every time we enter the room, she places her face very close to his, takes his large hand firmly in hers, and talks to him in a playful, yet respectful voice. On one occasion, she touches his hand to her nose in a sprightly affectionate gesture...and there it is — a tiny upward crease forming at the edge of his mouth. She has a reaction.

Jane habitually pinched her patient's big toe as she entered or left the room. When I asked her about it, she said, "I just do it to sort of lighten things up.... It's like a bit of fun in a rather serious place. I hope it relaxes them and lets them know it's still okay to play."

At other times, nurses used modifications of more conventional social touch such as the handshake to signify official acquaintance. Although a formal shaking of the hands was seldom observed, Maureen described how she introduces herself to patients.

> When I introduce myself, I go up and tell them my name and touch their hand lightly. It's like a handshake, only more. It formalizes our meeting for the first time, but it allows me to find out about them. Do they like to be touched, for example, or are they very apprehensive about being here?

In this way, the social touch serves more purposes for these nurses than a traditional recognition of the other. It is, in some ways, also a first assessment of the patient's needs and a communication to the patient that the nurse is willing to engage in mutual touching.

## Diagnostic touch

Through touch, nurses may "identify...body heat, discern skin textures, and recognize changes, favorable or unfavorable" in the patient's condition.[99] I have called touch that is primarily used for such purposes diagnostic touch.

The nurses I observed used their hands to assess the patient. For them, touch was an important means of discriminating between diagnoses. Several nurses talked about this important function of touch saying, "Feeling my patient's skin tells me a lot.... I touch them to see if they're cold, sweating, dry, or feverish." "I read my patient's status with my hands." "I have tested myself; I can tell a patient's temperature with almost perfect accuracy without using a thermometer." "I couldn't start an IV if I couldn't see the veins with my fingers."

How did they develop such an acute and accurate sense of touch? The consensus among the nurses I discussed this with was that they learned through experience. Lana said, "When I first started, I didn't know what hot was. Now that I have felt thousands of foreheads, I compare what I feel to what I know normal feels like." As the cited comments imply, diagnosis of a patient's physical status often comes to exceptionally competent nurses through their sense of touch.

### Comforting touch

Touching was a means used by these nurses to comfort their patients. Morse claims that the two major components of comfort are talking and touching. She explains, "Comfort measures vary according to situation, context, and meaning to each subject."[100] Depending on these factors, the nurse can choose to comfort a patient by talking, talking with a little touching, or touching with little talking. In Morse's opinion, all three approaches could comfort a patient.[101]

Benner recommends the use of touch in providing comfort, "Nurses frequently use touch to provide comfort and reach out to a withdrawn, depressed patient. Often, this human warm contact is the only avenue of comfort and communication available."[102] Montagu agrees and explains that "taking almost anyone's hand under conditions of stress is likely to exert a soothing effect, and by reducing anxiety it gives both the receiver and the giver a feeling of greater security."[103]

The nurses I interviewed were in agreement with these authors. Julie stated, "Our families in this society are so dispersed and alienated, the only way you get them comfort is through the touch of human kindness." Jane commented, "I think that a lot is communicated through touch. You can show concern...and break down a lot of barriers with touch. It affirms the patient as more than an object. It gives them the ultimate gift — comfort."

The use of touch and physical closeness may be important ways to communicate to acutely ill persons that they are important as human beings; yet critically ill patients are seldom touched by their caregivers in non-technical ways. Barriers created by the mechanical means used to support life may inhibit the use of human contact in providing comfort. A situation I observed provides an example of how the exemplary nurse worked around these impediments to bring the patient comfort.

> The patient is dwarfed by the obtrusiveness of the machines. On both sides of the bed, infusion pumps beep out their progress. Multiple bags of red-labeled solutions drip along, keeping time with the mechanical tones. Chest tube suction devices bubble and honk intrusively. Both side rails are in their upright position — the aim, to keep the patient in — the result, the world is kept out. The nurse walks up to the unresponsive patient and for a minute watches his shallow breathing. Then she reaches past the cumbersome array of machines and rests her hand on his still shoulder. As she leaves, she gently brushes a few strands of hair back off his forehead.

One day on the unit, Julie talked to me about how she uses touch to provide psychological comfort to the newly admitted patient. She said, "When a patient first comes through those doors, no matter how prepared they think they are, they really aren't. I try to establish some connection with them right away. Often it's just as simple as a little touch." Later she told this story.

> We had an HIV fellow with Kaposi's sarcoma, a new admission. I was going to help him with his meal. I didn't have any gloves on. This was his first supper with us and

he was totally coherent and a little anxious. I introduced myself and was giving him some help with his housecoat and he said, "You don't have any gloves on; aren't you scared?" I said, "Well, are you going to bite me?" He laughed and said, "No, but in the other hospital that I just came from, everyone wore gloves and gowns every time they came into my room." I just explained to him that, when I changed his dressings, I would wear gloves but that there was no medical reason to now, and I just kept helping him with his clothes.

I think I really made him feel comfortable — not that I even touched him that much at that moment, but I showed him I was willing to touch him. I don't think he had been touched by human hands that weren't covered in gloves for a long time. Touching him removed huge potential barriers between us and made him feel a lot less anxious.

In making this patient comfortable and comforted, the nurse felt more comfortable herself. Touching is a symbol of caring — a means to share feelings. It has a dual nature; we use it to comfort each other.

In another field note, I recorded how Jane comforted and calmed a patient who was struggling to breathe.

Even before we entered the room, I could hear the desperate gasps for air. As I laid my eyes on him, I could see his struggle. Starved for oxygen — physiologically by his disease, and psychologically by his mind — he fought for every breath. I watched as the nurse walked to his side and took his hand. In a very soft and reassuring voice, Jane said to him over and over, "Take it easy. Relax. Take it slower." Her repetitive words were

matched by repetitive stokes of his forearm. She was so
calm herself, and as his eyes fixed on hers, together they
slowed his breathing down until the desperation left.

—

**THE COMFORT OF A TOUCH**
Soothe, support, strengthen.
You can do it all with
just the perfect touch.

—

## The final touch

Many of the exemplary nurses expressed the belief that the sense
of touch is one of the last — perhaps the last — senses to leave the
dying person. The following field note illustrates how Maureen used
this type of touch.

> Sophia was dying. Life had become heavier than death.
> Her nurse was aware of her reality and visited her room
> often that day. Most times, there was no medical reason
> for her visits; she would just hold Sophia's hand and
> stroke her forehead. Sometimes she would pull up a chair
> and sit for a few minutes and read some of the get-well
> cards that Sophia could no longer see for herself. This
> seemed to be exactly what Sophia needed — someone
> who was willing to be near, to touch her gently.

The nurses agreed with Watson, who claims, "Patients who have no
apparent verbal capacity can usually feel a gentle touch and understand
its message of caring interest."[104] Because of this belief, the exceptional
nurses used touch, sometimes exclusively, in communicating with
patients during their last days. Maureen phrased it like this:

> I believe that when someone is dying they feel touch
> until the very end. I tell the family that, and I encourage

them to hold hands and stroke the patient's forehead. I do it too, just to let them know I am still with them.

Julie said,

> I use touch a lot when a patient is dying or has just died because I believe it is extremely important. I have found that the families watch you. When I go into a room just after a person has died, I always talk to the patient and say goodbye and I always touch them. It seems to make it okay for the rest of the family to do that. I have had a lot of positive feedback from families about it.

She then went on to tell me this story:

> A young man was dying — in a coma and totally non-responsive. I called his Mom and Dad (they lived out-of-town) and they arrived just in time for their son's dying day. I encouraged them to help me with his care, to touch him, and to talk to him. I got them chairs and coffee and checked in on them often. When I cared for him myself, I reminded him of the presence of his family, and I tried to set an example for them to follow.
>
> Near the end, they were doing really well and I witnessed something I will never forget. His Mom was washing his face — probably just like she had when he was a little boy. For just one short moment, he opened his eyes. He hadn't done that for many days. I know he saw her and she saw him. It was a wonderful moment, a last goodbye.

When I asked about her approach to caring for patients near death, Lana simply said, "I never leave a dying patient without a hand to hold." Several nurse researchers agree with this belief that touch is important in the last hours of life. Chang contends that a great many needs of terminal patients will be satisfied non-verbally through empathetic nursing care.[105] The psychological impact of non-verbal communication, especially of touch, on the dying patient cannot be underrated. Watson, agreeing with this point, reports that "our first contact with life is through touch as an infant...our first comfort in life comes from touch and usually our last. Through touch we may communicate with comatose, dying patients when words have no way of breaking through."[106]

A story written by Marie illustrates that the use of touch in the final moments is effective even if the nurse is unfamiliar with the patient and family.

It was a busy shift. I had been away on holidays for a month, and this was my first shift back. The only patients I knew on the ward were the six I was assigned to. It was about 2100 hours, and I needed a dressing tray so I was walking quickly towards the clean utility room to get one. The hallways were darkened, and as I walked by a patient's room, I was grabbed by the arm by a visitor beckoning me. "Nurse, please come," he said. I entered the room of a patient who was taking his last breaths. He ceased breathing and I looked up at the faces surrounding me. "Is he gone?" asked a younger man, presumably his son. "Yes," was all I could think of to say.

I felt so inadequate at that moment; I didn't know his name, the family, or the previous circumstances. I stumbled, "I'm so sorry," and sat down with them holding onto a hand and a shoulder. I knew I was needed by my own patients, but this moment demanded every inch of me now. I noticed how peacefully he died so I shared that with the family, and they shared a few memories with me. For those few initial moments, we mostly just sat and held hands. It was like they needed a nurse present for this rite of passage. Soon, the patient's nurse arrived, and I scurried down the hall realizing I had a dressing to do.

When I talked to Marie later about this episode, she offered further insights. She said,

> This man was taking his last breaths. All I could do was bring his family closer and put their hands on him while I supported them. I realized afterwards how quickly we move in and out of people's lives. I did not know their names, but that short interlude was strengthening to me. I was needed, and I also received. I think it was touching that allowed us to make an intense connection in a very short time. Nurses seem to have the right, and privilege, to touch people — even people who were complete strangers moments before. Touch is one of the most important ways I communicate.

—

**THE UNKNOWN PATIENT**

You call for a nurse,
and the nurse in me instinctively responds.

You are alone and afraid
in this moment of need.
I don't know you,
yet you are so familiar to me.
I sense your anguish, your uncertainty.

Hand in hand we unite our spirits
and send your loved one on his journey.

—

## TOUCH AND SILENCE

Touch and silence have many similarities. Although they need not always be companions, touch seems to be a natural complement to silence. Like the dialogue of silence, mutual touch is a non-verbal form of inter-human communication. Touch shares a further similarity to silence in that both affect the sender and the receiver, the toucher and the touched.

Touch, like silence, can be effective in both emotionally demanding circumstances and during everyday patient encounters. Both touch and silence were used to communicate and receive messages, feelings, and emotions that would be difficult to share in any other way. Touch and silence both facilitate the sharing of emotions.

Comparing further, messages sent through silence and touch involve the similarity of instantaneousness. That is, messages embedded in silence and touch are received as they are sent. There is usually no delay. Both participants can send and receive understandings at the same time, making these two modes of communication efficient.

Unspoken messages are embedded in touch and silent exchanges — messages that may give the patient comfort and humanize the situation. Although silence and touch are often only a part of a nursing intervention, they are components that seem important in exceptional nursing practice.

———

**THE IMPRINT**
Your touch.
A gentle brush across my cheek.
How can something so faint,
so soft,
so subtle,
leave such an indelible imprint
on our souls?

———

# *chapter five*

SHARING THE LIGHTER SIDE
OF LIFE

*A merry heart doeth good like a medicine;*
*but a broken spirit drieth the bones.*[107]

This chapter focuses on the third theme in the trilogy, sharing the lighter side of life. A lighthearted attitude is common among the exemplary nurses. Despite tragic circumstances in their work lives, most times these nurses deliberately choose to see the positive and humorous side of situations. Importantly, they are able to share this orientation to life effectively and appropriately with their colleagues and patients.

The literature often refers to this approach in a narrow sense, labeling it the deliberate therapeutic use of humour. Intentional attempts to introduce humour 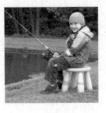 into patient care using comic videos, cartoons, jokes, and clowns are recommended by several writers.[108-111] Although excerpts from the literature are included in this chapter to augment the discussion, this theme goes well beyond the staged use of humour in nursing care. As Thomas says, using humour is more than the presence of a nurse who is a stand-up comedian or an entertainer.[112]

The fifth chapter has four major sections: a definition of this lighthearted attitude, the functions of humour (the communication, social, psychological, and therapeutic purposes); different forms of humour (surprise, word play, black, situational, and divergent); and a comment on developing a lighthearted attitude.

Poems are incorporated into the text of the chapter. The nurses' words and my field notes illustrate the theme. In this chapter, the narratives are especially detailed because, as Benner and Wrubel caution, "Humor is not easily understood out of context.... It is specific to the situation and easily misunderstood."[113]

## THE LIGHTHEARTED ATTITUDE DEFINED

Defining an attitude is difficult. Robinson pointed out that it is as difficult to find a universal definition of the term *humour* as it is to achieve a universal language.[114] In my attempt to describe what is meant by a lighthearted attitude I address four topics in this section: the part that humour and laughter play in this orientation, what such an attitude may look like, the element of choice, and the role of this orientation to life when circumstances are tragic.

### *Humour and laughter*

Thomas contends that defining humour is like "tacking jelly to the wall."[115] Humour is an elusive concept. Originally, the term meant a liquid that flowed within the body controlling one's health and disposition. Physicians attempted to keep people in "good humour." Humour continues to be considered in part as an internal condition, as in one's sense of humour.

Astedt-Kurki and Liukkonen define humour as *joie de vivre*, which is manifested in human interaction in the form of fun, jocularity and laughter.[116] They acknowledge that humour is a complex cognitive and emotional process. Hunt establishes that humour can be "many things to many people," that it must be interpreted, and that it is "whatever people think is funny."[117] Baughman identifies humour as our sixth sense, as important as any of the other five. He writes,

Much more should be said and written about humor, for so many think it means no more than the ability to tell a funny story or to respond to one. Actually, a sense of humor refers to a complete philosophy of life. It includes the ability to take it as well as to hand it out. It includes poise, the capacity to bend without breaking, taking life's responsibilities seriously but oneself not too seriously. Other less obvious components of humor are these: the ability to relax, to escape from tension, to get pleasure out of the joys of others, to live unselfishly, laughing with people.[118]

This broad definition of humour is congruent with the attitude displayed by the nurses in the study. However, laughter, though often the result of humour, is viewed in the literature as different from humour. Thomas defines laughter as a bodily response to things that are both humorous and not so.[119] Lefcourt and Martin suggest it is "a reflex-like physiologic-behavioral response."[120]

Many of the exceptional nurses commented that laughter does not necessarily follow a humorous incident. As Julie explained, "Sometimes when a situation is really awful, all you can do is laugh. We had a family member who giggled as a reaction to tense situations. He just couldn't deal with what was happening. Especially when it wasn't funny, he would laugh."

Humour and laughter are a part of sharing the lighter side of life, but this attitude goes further. It is an all-encompassing disposition, an ability to see the lighter side of situations and encounters as they occur. It is a daily, moment by moment alertness to the possibility of seeing the funny, the humorous, and the laughable — even in the most unhappy and desperate moments. This spirit of lightness served as a lens through which the exemplary nurses viewed their worlds, and through which they helped others to see their own worlds differently.

What does it mean to see the lighter side of life? It is a state of mind in which the humorous, the bizarre, and the less traumatic are seen in the events of life and responded to in a lighthearted way. A sensitivity to life's lighter side involves spontaneity, lightheartedness, and an ability to play — all of which are needed for humour to occur. As Leacock said, it is "seeing the fun of the thing."[121]

## Qualities of a lighthearted attitude

How does one recognize a lighthearted attitude in another person? The nurses I observed and talked to displayed this orientation to life in a variety of ways. Part of it was non-verbal. Their physical appearance, the way they dressed, moved, and used gestures, signaled that they were positive, energetic people, open to sharing their vitality. These descriptions of some of the nurses from my field notes illustrate this attitude:

- She is bubbly, full of energy and lustrous smiles. Today she is wearing a bright peach uniform and a name tag that is far from ordinary.

- This morning she greeted me with a big, genuine smile. The multi-colored smock that she wore over her whiter-than-white uniform made me notice her.

- Her arms move in time with her words; her steps are never hesitant. She is open, uses direct eye contact, laughs easily, and proclaims, "I can't be phony."

- His approach is playful and full of fun — yet very respectful. Looking into his eyes, you see life.

- She smiles a lot. I am at once attracted by her energy and vitality. She is someone I want to be around. It's hard to put into words, but she is somewhat like a magnet — attracting me, pulling me to her.

A second part of their positive view of life was shared through the verbal components of their nursing care. The delivery of their comments, including the timing of presentation, was important in communicating this attitude. In one field note I wrote, "The quality of her voice, the cadence and rhythm of her speech — all communicate this sense of zest for life."

Peter was especially effective at incorporating playful comments into his patient care activities. As he was helping a patient put on his pants without success, he would say, "Maybe we should try to get one leg in each hole." While handing out menus on which the patients would mark their meal choices, he would smile and remark, "Here's your homework for today." These little side comments and the buoyant way they were delivered always made the patients smile.

## Choosing to see humour in difficult situations

Looking on the bright side of life is a conscious decision that, in time, becomes a habit. Julie modeled this belief. She felt that every person has a choice about how they view the events of life. One story she wrote ended this way: "Every day is a mixture of good and bad. No day is 100 percent good or bad. But you will have good or bad days depending on your focus." When I asked her about the origin of this attitude, she told me about a statue that she had seen in New York city. It was a cage, and inside was a pregnant woman with several children clinging to her skirts. The caption read, "We build our own cages." Julie elaborated, saying,

> We are empowered to make choices and, unfortunately, we get into situations where our horizons are the edges of the ruts that we dig for ourselves. When that happens, we can't see to either side or the light at the end of the tunnel. It takes the fun out of things. If we just realize we have alternatives as to how we see life, we can breathe.

Jane wrote, "One's perspective makes all the difference in whether or not any experience is transcending, transforming, depressing, or devastating to the people involved."

Marie said, "When I was thinking of stories to write for you, I found that many of the most significant made me chuckle." This humour affected the way the nurses perceived and performed their work. The following stories are examples of how the nurses chose to see the humour in unusual patient encounters.

There was this male patient — he was in isolation so no one could go into his room unless it was really necessary. Often, I would just stop by the door of his room to say "Hi" and see how he was doing.

On one visit, he mentioned he was cold. I said I would try to get help, but it was unlikely a repair man could go in to fix his radiator. He smiled and said, "Not a problem — I happen to be a repair man myself." I jokingly said, "Do what you can," and left.

The next time I walked by his room, I peeked in and he had the whole radiator panel off. Parts of the radiator were on the floor. I said, "What are you doing?" He answered, "I've got it under control." What could I do? He was so happy, passing the time; his hands were full of grease and he was smiling. So I just said, "That's great — but we won't be paying you." By the time he was discharged, it was all cleaned up and until now it has been our secret.

Mrs. Ling really helped me appreciate cultural differences and to see how some cultures clash with the hospital culture in a funny way. I don't know why, but Mrs. Ling really liked me. I didn't even speak Chinese or anything.

To show her appreciation to me, one day when I went into her room she pulled out these long, slimy, red ginseng roots. She said, "Is good. You eat it." I took it and smiled, and slipped it into my cheek as I stepped out of the room. I didn't eat it. I just kept hoping that she was right — that it was ginseng. When I think of it, even at the time I saw the humour in it. What a funny sight we must have been — this tiny elderly woman giving me this great "gift" and me trying to stuff this "worm" into my cheek without gagging, all the while maintaining a look of sincere gratitude. I just had to do it because I thought it was probably really important to her. She probably loves the stuff, and she had it saved for me. It was a symbol of her gratitude. It still makes me laugh when I think of it.

I was calling this "gentleman" patient for seven consecutive days at home. He was on a research protocol, and as part of the procedure, I had to phone him and find out how he was doing with his medication and what his pain level was. He was just a really coarse sort of guy — you know, he had frayed edges. When I'd call he'd say, "How the hell do you think I am? I'm not taking this damn stuff anymore." When I'd ask about his pain level, it would always be ten out of ten.

One night when I had to call him, I was not at the hospital; I was at the local fair and exhibition. The only phone I could find was in a saloon. Phoning him was the last thing I wanted to do. When I called, he characteristically said, "Where the hell are you — at a bar or something?" I said, "You are right; I'm at a saloon." At the time, he was shocked, but we laughed about it together even a day later. I heard that he died, but I was happy that I had this wonderful memory of him. It wasn't tender. We were never close, and we certainly never touched each other — but maybe I touched him with my humour, and he did touch me with his.

Sarah was a Native woman from the reserve. She hadn't been to the city many times, and now she had to be hospitalized and was totally overwhelmed by the whole thing. She was my patient, and she had to go for a diagnostic test. I had to get her ready to go. She didn't know English, and I didn't know Cree, but I did my best to demonstrate what would be happening to her. She finally understood that she had to take her clothes off and go to the procedure wearing just a hospital gown. I just smiled every time I went to her room. She was just a joy to me. No teeth, beaded moccasins, skin of leather — she had really lived the tipi life.

The vision I have is of me trying to coax this woman onto a stretcher to go for the procedure. Here I am — a white woman — coming into her room, demanding her clothes, and trying to give her an injection in her buttocks. It was just against her whole tradition, her whole culture; it was just too much for her.

In a swift decisive move, Sarah jumped off the stretcher and ran in her moccasin slippers down the hall. Most of the staff were running after her. I was trying to stay calm, saying to myself, "You can handle this," but another part of me was just so tickled by her spunk. I was cheering, "Way to go Sarah!"

In these and similar situations, the nurses' inclination might have been to react in a negative way — becoming upset or angry. However, the nurses in the stories were open to seeing the humour in the incidents. At the moment the event occurred, and later as they recalled the situations, they chose to see the lighter side.

—

**MAINTAINING THE ATTITUDE**

When things are going well,
it's easy to keep the rhythm in your step,
the enthusiasm on your face,
and the shine in your eyes.

But when life gets challenging,
ordinary people lose it.
You don't.

—

*Appropriateness of humour in a tragic environment*

The sage Epictetus says it is not the things that happen that distresses people, it is their opinion about the things that happen. Olsson, Backe, Sorensen, and Kock agreed saying that, in most tragic conditions and adverse environments, being sad and heavy yourself adds to the unhappiness.[122]

If a lighthearted attitude is a method for survival, it is not surprising that humour and laughter were present on the cancer unit. Nurses who work in stressful environments may need to joke and laugh to cope with the seriousness found there. Feelings that are too painful to deal with can be put on hold or eased by humour. Benner and Wrubel share this view and add, "Humor is used to establish rapport and alter situations of grave seriousness and despair."[123] Recent research by Dean and Major also found that life-threatening circumstances and high anxiety are times when humour may be appropriate.[124] They conclude that humour in these situations enables co-operation, relieves tensions, develops emotional flexibility and "humanizes" the healthcare experience for both caregivers and recipients of care.[125]

In the same vein, McDougall writes, "Humor was devised so that we would not be overwhelmed by the misfortunes of life. We are inclined to sympathize too much, and we would be devastated if we did not have an antidote. Laughter is that antidote."[126]

If we accept Baughman's views on humour, it is understandable why humour is appropriate and important in an oncology setting. Baughman proclaims, "Humor is that soothing and compensating piece of mind which prevents us from being overcome by life's adversities. It can dissipate the fog and make life more enjoyable and far less threatening."[127] Agreeing with this view, Yura and Walsh note that humour can create a warm climate, promote good interpersonal relationships, and relieve feelings of frustration, anxiety, or hostility while helping nurses and patients achieve a broader perspective on life.[128] Some humour may actually arise out of turmoil and anguish. Humour is a means of addressing all that is imperfect in the human condition.

In one of my first field notes I wrote,

> I am surprised by the amount of teasing, joking, and laughter here — not just among the nurses, but with the patients, too. I just didn't expect it in an environment that has so much potential to be dark and depressing. Somehow humour and laughter decrease the gloom and replace it with a sense of merriment.

Cindy told me, "There is always laughter on this unit. It's important for all of us. Some patients say hearing the laughter makes it human here."

As I continued to collect data, my first impression was confirmed. Three nurses explained why it is important to their success to see and share the lighter side of life.

I enjoy sharing laughter and do it a lot. I'll see a situation and then inject the absurd into it, just to get a laugh. It's especially important here because people can be stressed and depressed. Laughter sets people at ease. It gives them permission to be spontaneous — to be themselves. It tells suffering people that it's okay to smile.

It's normal and natural to laugh.... It's abnormal not to, even in a place like this.

Laughing is important in our situation because it can be so sad. In my experience, there is a close relationship between tears and laughter.

---

**INTERSECTING LINES**
Looking into the woman's face
I could see the lines intersecting,
lines of laughter and lines of despair,
criss-crossing to form a pattern on her skin.

The way they came together so naturally,
it was apparent they had met often before.

---

Sharing the lighter side of life on a cancer unit requires impeccable sensitivity and tact on the part of the nurse. Julie commented,

We use humour delicately. It requires a careful matching of types of humour with specific patients and situations. I consider it carefully. I think, "What kind of humour would this patient like — or would they be open to it at all?" When you use humour is important too. Timing is critical.

As Hunt cautions, "Individuals have differences in what they experience as humor. Individuals also have religious preferences, cultural experiences, and unique values that make certain kinds of humor unacceptable."[129] He continues by saying, "Careful nursing assessment [should] be done prior to utilizing humor … like any other intervention strategy, there are indications for, limits to, and contraindications for the use of humor."[130] Pasquali warns that humour is inappropriate when it ignores client humour styles, ridicules, or is racist or sarcastic.[131]

Jane observed, "When using humour it is important to determine what is appropriate and what is not. I am very careful when the patient is in pain, suffering, confused, or depressed. At these times, it might not be helpful to laugh or be playful." Blondis and Jackson agree and caution, "When using humor, use not only what is comfortable for you, but what is acceptable to the other person."[132] To be effective, humour must be appropriate to the audience and the situation.

In summary, a definition of this approach to life reveals that, although humour and laughter are part of a lighthearted attitude, this attitude goes beyond these elements and is more complex and comprehensive in nature. It includes both verbal and non-verbal components, enactment is a deliberate choice, and it can be appropriate in difficult circumstances if it is used with sensitivity.

### THE VALUE OF SHARING LIGHTNESS

It appears a lighthearted attitude serves at least three therapeutic purposes: communication is enhanced, a social purpose is achieved, and it has psychological value.

*Communication*

Leacock concluded, "But most of all, we laugh."[133] Humour, laughter, and a lighthearted attitude were used by the nurses to communicate important messages to the patients. Lana said, "When you have this kind of approach to life — where you see the positive in things — you laugh easily, and smile a lot; it tells patients you are a person who is willing to share their lives, their troubles, their joys."

Maureen shared a memory as an example of such a message:

> Jerry had been diagnosed with acute leukemia for over a year. As with most patients who receive many courses of chemotherapy, we had developed a strong relationship with Jerry and his wife. Jerry was originally from Scotland and spoke with a thick Scottish accent. He referred to all the nurses as "sweetheart," and that was fine with us. His sense of humour was always present and he was quick to share a joke with a receptive person.
>
> Jerry was in remission and was supposed to have a potentially life-saving bone marrow transplant in Toronto. However, his brother, who was expected to be the donor, was found to have incompatible marrow. The transplant, his last hope for a long and healthy life, was cancelled.
>
> This was his first admission since his disappointing trip to Toronto, and the nursing staff were unsure of how to approach him. I was no different, and walking down the hall to his room was one of the most difficult walks I have made. I took a deep breath and entered his room. He was the first to acknowledge my presence. "Hi, sweetheart," he said. "I'm back." I looked at him, smiled, and said, "Don't tell me, Jerry — the nurses in Toronto didn't laugh at your jokes so you had to come home."
>
> With that Jerry started to laugh. "You're right," he said. "I missed you girls." That was all it took to break the tension. At that point, I sat next to him on his bed and listened as he told me of his trip, his disappointment, and his hopes for the future.

—

**ENTERING YOUR EXPERIENCE**
Shared laughter
is a conduit into your experience.
It rivets us together,
so for an instant
we understand.

—

Maureen said about laughing with a patient,

I think it signals to the patients that you have time for them — time for more than the nursing procedures I mean. If you joke around with them, it means you value them. They are worthy of your time and attention.

Humour was sometimes used by the nurses when the messages to be communicated were very serious and emotion-laden. In these situations, the direct expression would have been uncomfortable for both the nurse and patient. In the following scenario, taken from my field notes, the lighthearted approach was used to communicate information indirectly. Though the meaning was concealed, the patient understood.

It was late at night and a distraught patient rang her bell and asked the nurse I was observing for an anti-anxiety medication. After assessing the situation, the nurse determined that such a medication would not be appropriate in this patient's circumstances because it could hasten death. To communicate this message to the patient, the nurse gently said, "Mrs. James, I'm afraid to give you the pill you asked for because it would make you sleep — sleep too long." For a moment there was silence, and then the patient understood this delicately worded message and they both smiled knowingly.

Outside the room Julie offered this analysis of the situation.

> I believe in always telling patients the truth, but some-
> times it's just too brutal to say it outright. What was I
> supposed to say to her — "If I give you the pill you want,
> it will probably kill you?" I just couldn't put it that way.
> The lighthearted approach is better — especially when
> the topic is such a heavy one.

—

**THE MOURNFUL LAUGH**
Sometimes
the topics that are the most
laughable
are those that are so somber and sad
that ordinary words can't do them justice.

—

"Laughter," Moria said, "almost always precedes the tears. It somehow opens the gateway, allowing for meaningful communication of
the real issues." Moody puts it this way: "Humour is an important
pass key into an environment in which the locks are always changing."[134] Clearly, a lighthearted approach can enhance the communication function.

## Social Purpose

Sharing the lighter moments is part of creating a bond between the
nurse and patient. As Jane said,

> When you spend time with your patients laughing and
> joking together, it tells them that you want to share
> something of yourself with them — and you get to know
> another part of them, too. This makes you friends in a
> way. It gives a sense of solidarity.

Dean and Major support this belief as they emphasize that humour helps establish relationships.[135] The value of humour resides, not in its capacity to alter physical reality, but in its capacity for affective or psychological change which enhances the humanity of an experience. In particular, they point to the value of humour for teamwork, emotion management, and maintaining human connections. Julie commented, "You are acknowledging a person when you laugh appropriately. You are saying, 'Yes, I understand what you are saying.'"

Julie shared the following story, which illustrates the social bonding that can occur between nurse and patient and the patient's family members through humour.

I enjoy laughing with my patients, but one of my unforgettable moments began by being laughed at. The patient was newly admitted. He did not want to be here; he wanted to die at home. After all, he owned a funeral home and he knew about dying. He seemed to have a dozen children. They really didn't want him here either. Each was dealing with their guilt and hurt in their own way. The room was always packed with people, but it was not necessarily a friendly place to be.

When I walked in, the hostility was acrid, but my name tag said "nurse" and that gave me license to be there. Besides, the man was definitely end stage, and it would have been totally wrong for him to die without even having his blood pressure recorded! So in a feeble attempt to give him care, that's what I did; I took his pressure.

As my stethoscope was plugging my ears, I only picked up pieces of a conversation that was occurring in the room around me. "I don't think she could walk this far." "Maybe they have visiting hours." "She's old, you know — and so fat."

Having finally found his blood pressure and wanting to make a significant contribution to the overheard puzzle pieces, I very innocently said, "I couldn't help overhearing. If there's anything we can do to help with the visit, we would be glad to. We have wheelchairs. Feel free to borrow one."

Whereupon the room was filled to overflowing with gales of laughter. One fellow even fell weak-kneed into a chair. Tissues that once held tears of sadness were now wiping away drops of hilarity. It turned out the elderly, crippled, maiden aunt that I had envisioned was an old arthritic, overweight English bulldog who probably wouldn't have even fit in the wheelchair!!

Yes, the dog did visit. In fact, she monopolized the patient's bed, by this time far outweighing her cachexic master. There were many more smiles and yes, many more tears — both happy and sad — but the bond created by the original faux pas remained strong.

—

**SOCIAL CLIMATE CHANGE**
Laughing together
makes the social climate,
summer or winter,
ideal.

—

I watched the exemplary nurses use humour and playfulness in their actions and voices to help them build relationships almost instantly with patients. On one occasion, as we entered the room of a new patient carrying a bag of intravenous solution, the nurse said, "Hi, I'm your nurse — the bag lady." The patient and visitors laughed because this well-dressed, poised, carefully groomed woman was obviously not a bag lady. My field note reads, "They laughed together at the absurdity of the comment and, as they laughed, the tension in the room eased and the door was opened for important serious exchanges."

The literature also suggests that sharing humour helps establish relationships and aids in creating rapport.[136] Julie talked about this outcome when she said,

> There is a sense of cohesion that develops when you share inside jokes with someone. I do this with my patients and also with the other staff members. For example, we have certain abbreviations that we use that no one else knows the meaning of, like FOS and PON. When we say these code words in report, it makes us laugh — it makes us a team, special somehow because only we know the meaning.

Both the caregivers and the patients are initiators of humour, especially for social purposes. Jane told me she gives her patients permission to joke and laugh by her example. She remembered with delight one patient who followed her lead.

> He rang his bell, and when I asked him how I could help, he said, "Well, I just washed my hair and I can't do a thing with it." It was really funny because he only had one or two hairs left; he had lost almost all of his hair from chemotherapy. We both laughed. At that moment I felt very close to him, and I am sure he could tell that I cared.

Julie said, "The patients really seem to enjoy the atmosphere around here. They tell us jokes sometimes. The other day, one man told me the rankest joke; it was so bad I really didn't understand it — but it made us laugh."

Baughman describes humour as a "social lubricant."[137] It eases social situations and promotes smooth and comfortable social interaction. Humour helps to establish relationships, decrease fears, encourage trust, increase the feeling of friendship, and decrease the social distance as it invites others to come close.

In observing embarrassing moments and errors made, I noticed that humour was often used to "lubricate" these situations. For example, one day in the unit Cindy discovered that a patient had not been assigned a nurse and had gone through part of the day without care. The nurse who had made the error was remorseful. Instead of becoming angry or agitated, Cindy just said, "I guess God had him this morning." The situation was resolved; no harm had come to the patient, and a lesson was learned while the light atmosphere was maintained. Dean and Major suggest that humour helps resolve potentially disastrous social interactions by trivializing potentially serious incidents and helping one save face.[138]

I observed nurses using humour when carrying out procedures that were potentially embarrassing or humiliating for the patient. In one instance, Julie had just given a very small, fragile, shy man an enema which had been very effective. The patient was uncomfortable with the process until Julie lightened the scene when she exclaimed, "Why, Mr. Godfree, I didn't know you weighed that much." On a similar occasion, she said to the patient with a smile, "You done good, buddy."

Nurses who exhibit this sense of lightheartedness convey to others a warmth, friendliness, and acceptance. This probably affects how others perceive them. It makes them seem real, human, and approachable — the kind of people you chose to trust with your problems and feelings.

Dean and Major describe qualities of humour that make it important in effective caregiver-patient interaction.[139] Humour allows the nurse to probe, to find out more about the patient's feelings and fears without taking real risk. In this way, humour has an unmasking quality. According to these authors, humour moves people toward intimacy; it is an invitation to interact on a more personal level.[140]

—

**FUNNY THING ABOUT LAUGHTER**
When we laugh together,
it somehow shortens the distance between us,
it reduces the space we occupy,
but doesn't make it
any more crowded.

—

## Psychological Value

Baughman quipped, "Humour is like a diaper change. It doesn't solve any problems permanently. It just makes life a bit more comfortable for awhile."[141] Humour itself is one of the good things of life. Humour in relationships can release tension and create a moment of positivity. To dispense laughter to someone would be to increase the quality of this life.[142] Humour animates and provides a change of pace. For these reasons, and others, sharing the lighter side of life offers a psychological value for patients and staff.

Exemplary nurses believe that sharing moments of lightness helps to comfort patients. Both the nurses and the patients commonly exchanged old jokes that had long since ceased being funny. The patients would say, "I suppose you are going to wake me up to give me a sleeping pill," or the nurse would jest, "You must be feeling like a pin cushion," and both the patients and nurses would laugh. There is some comfort in laughing at these tired jokes. It is analogous to putting on well-worn slippers; it just feels good. If one is still laughing at the same routine, this signals that things are fine, that nothing has changed. Perhaps it is important that they are old jokes and their familiarity is a comfort.

Lightheartedness can also act as a safety value — a mechanism used to release stress. Baughman explains how this happens: "Laughter eases aggression, anger, and distress by taking one's mind off the situation at hand by casting a different interpretation of life."[143]

Lana, in describing how laughter eased the tension in a situation she encountered said, "Somehow, even a little titter decreases the intensity of the moment and makes it so we can carry on." This effect of humour was demonstrated by a nurse-patient encounter I witnessed and recorded.

> I was watching as the nurse was trying to talk a patient into having a bath she was refusing to take. The nurse had used a variety of approaches aimed at persuading the patient that a bath was in her best interest. At the precise moment when the scene could have become uncomfortable for the patient, nurse, and visitors, the nurse said, "That's the problem with nurses. If all else fails, we wash it." Everyone laughed, the tension eased, and the woman consented to the bath.

During another conversation, Julie told me this story about laughter easing tension.

> Sometimes the responses I get are more expressions of shock from the patients, but it really relieves the tension when you can get a laugh. Yesterday I was looking around for some tube sites on this fellow. The records hadn't been updated, so I didn't know for sure where on his body the tubes could be found. As I fumbled around peeking inside his pajama tops and bottoms I said, "I

think you should put me up for sexual harassment." The patient laughed and I enjoyed it. It put a lightness into the situation. It covered my incompetence and I think — no, I know — it made the patient more comfortable with what I was doing.

A lighthearted attitude also helps to develop an environment that is warm and nurturing, which is a psychological benefit. It also inspires hope. Moria indicated, "I think the patients like it when we laugh with them. I think they believe that, if we are still laughing, everything is still okay. It is reassuring; it gives them hope." As Lana said, "A sense of playfulness opens up discussion, breaks the cycle of despair, and fosters hope — because if you can laugh, you are still alive."

A classic humorist, Bradford, wrote,

> Humor not only brightens, it cleanses the common life. It is always on the side of hope, high hope. It is always on the side of promise. It asserts that the sun still shines, however dismal the weather of the moment, that the morning birds still sing, and what is more, that there is something to sing about.[144]

A lighthearted attitude helps to relieve anxiety and tension. It is a positive outlet for frustration and lightens the heaviness of critical situations. Jane commented, "When we laugh, it lightens the moment; it provides balance and hope." She called her attitude her "survival kit."

Humour can be an important part of caring for clients, caring for other nurses, and caring for ourselves. On one occasion in the field, the nurse I was observing, Julie, had encountered a novice nurse performing a procedure incorrectly. She had intervened to prevent danger to the patient and, in doing so, had caused the other nurse some personal embarrassment and distress. Later that shift, Julie used humour to re-establish connections with her young colleague. My field note reads,

> For the second time tonight, we come across a novice having trouble with technology. This time, she can't get an infusion pump to start. As we approach her, apprehension is apparent. She doesn't want to make another mistake and her anxiety makes her fumble inappropriately with the machine. Julie gently gives guidance saying, "Press A, then B — and it helps if you say the right prayer." She follows the directions, and the machine starts running. Julie smiles and says, "See, you must have said just the right prayer." They both laugh and the young nurse is able to carry on.

———

**THE FORGIVING LAUGH**
It is hard for you to laugh with me
and still carry your anger.
Your smile tells me in such a clear way
that I have been reinstated,
that I am once again your friend.

———

On another occasion, a nurse that Julie was supervising reported an error she had made. Julie just smiled and said, "That's okay. We try harder than most. But who can we blame? At times like this, it is nice to have someone to blame. It must have been the wandering nurse." During that shift the "wandering nurse" became the scapegoat for a variety of problems, including noxious odours and misplaced coffee cups.

I asked Julie about this situation in a conversation. She explained,

You have to know which things to deal with seriously, and which situations you can let go. That wasn't an error worth making a big deal about...so I made a joke out of it. It made her feel much better, and I know she learned more than she would have if I'd given her the big lecture.

A lighthearted attitude helps one meet unexpected events in the course of life. It can be a tonic that invigorates and stimulates those who share laughter. The nurses provided examples of this effect of humour and laughter; they argued that it provides refreshment and restoration for them as well as for the patients. Marie said, "Laughter in a room just fills the room with energy." Jane commented, "Laughter makes the world less drab somehow, and more human — much more human." Gruner agrees, "Human societies treasure laughter and whatever can produce it. Without laughter, everyday living becomes drab and lifeless; life would seem hardly human at all without it."[145]

In summary, Baughman explains the therapeutic function of humour in this way: "It creates happiness, fosters friendship, cheers the discouraged, and dissolves tensions. And as a bonus, it frees the mind, oils the squeaks, and enables us to carry on with fewer dark hours."[146]

—

**THE VALUE OF A LAUGH**

Laughter turns on the lights.

It is a defense against

panic,

sorrow,

and darkness and

it helps tide us over

until dawn.

—

## HUMOUR COMES IN MANY FORMS

What is humour? Why do we laugh? There are descriptions of several different forms of humour in the literature. Many of these forms of humour were observed during my field work. Surprise humour, word play, black or gallows humour, humour intrinsic to the situation, and divergent humour were some of the common forms.

As mentioned earlier, the nurses attempt to match their style of humour to what the patient appreciates. Jane said, "I change my style of humour to suit the person. I just push the buttons until I get a genuine response." In a field note, I wrote, "She takes her humour cues from others as to the type of humour that is suitable, and then improvises." Julie explained,

> I probably read them quite quickly. It depends, but I usually try it out when I am alone with them rather than when their families are there because the families may be shocked if I am too familiar. The families are tense, especially at the beginning. I usually use humour after the patient has been here for a while.

### Surprise humour

Marie often used surprise in her approach to humour. In this style, surprise, shock, or the unexpected are conditions necessary for humour. This story depicts Marie's use of a surprise style.

> My brand of humour is usually nice and dry, kind of subtle. This patient I am remembering was diagnosed with a head and neck cancer. He had a history of alcohol abuse. He was impossible. I guess I got the short straw at assignment time, and he was all mine. He was gruff, rude, verbally abusive — a real gem. What's more, he required trach. care, suctioning, and instillations. A perfect nurse-patient bonding activity.

I remember tiptoeing into his room, hoping he'd sleep through my evening shift. Hardly — he was waiting for me in dire need of suctioning, since he probably refused care from the respiratory therapist on days. Using humour was far from my mind at first. There was nothing he was going to find humorous, and I knew it. I was very professional with him, and I scraped by for two shifts. But, I had seven consecutive evening shifts scheduled, and I realized for the sake of patient–nurse continuity he should be mine for all seven evenings.

By the third shift, we had become more familiar with each other. I thought I'd try it. When I entered the room, I said, "Oh no — not you again," and rolled my eyes. I think my approach shocked him. He didn't expect a statement like that from such a "professional" nurse. Soon, he mimicked my actions, rolling his eyes when I entered his room. By the fifth shift, he broke into a smile, and I got a wink of the eye by the sixth. He and I were eager to see each other by my last shift and shared a few jokes. He did, in fact, request my care in future trach. procedures. Ah, this I count as success!

In another incident where surprise was used, a patient called the nurse, Jane, into his room. When she entered his room, his usually bald head was covered in a curly, long, blond woman's wig. The patient looked at the nurse and said, "Notice anything different?" The element of shock and surprise caused them to laugh together for a long time.

Finally, Maureen told me a story in which her own shock response to the patient helped to dissipate the patient's anger.

A patient slipped and fell on the floor. She overheard one of the nurses commenting that it happened at shift change. The patient got upset thinking that, because of the timing of the fall — at change of shift — the nurses might have ignored her there on the floor until report was over and the replacement nurses were on duty.

Well, I went and talked to her, and basically for half an hour I just listened to what she had to say and acknowledged that it was upsetting to think she might have been left on the floor. Then we started talking about other things, and I leaned over to her and said, "Next time, just make sure you don't fall at shift change!" She just started really laughing. Over the half hour, I figured out that she was quite a character and I knew she would respond to that kind of humour.

## Word play humour

Jane used word play, rhyming words, and lines from songs when providing care. These were a natural additive to her conversations with patients and others. Talking to a patient one day about his diarrhea, she rhymed, "It's just like the musical fruit, down your leg and into your boot." Entering a patient's room to bring him his noon meal, she said, "How would you like a bunch of lunch to munch and crunch?" Her poems and quips did not necessarily fit the context precisely, but the lyrical cadence of her voice was playful and reassuring.

## Black humour

Black humour was used often among staff members — usually in places that were isolated from the patients and family members. During team conferences, in the medication room, and during report, nurses and other care providers found a release of tension through humour that was dark and bizarre. Maureen explained, "The staff often use black humour — in the med. room especially. We would never, ever share what we talk about in there with the patients." For example, a physician was observed seriously advising the nurse who was caring for a man whose colostomy just would not stop, that he had ordered the same patient two doses of laxative. In another situation, Moria advised her teammates in jest that she was going home early today because "all of her patients were in the morgue." In fact, two of the four patients assigned to her care had died that day.

A field note provides a further example of the staff using black humour.

> A Catholic priest stopped to tell the nurse in charge, Julie, that the patient he had been called to see did not wish to see him because he was Catholic. Julie dead-panned, "I suppose she just swore at you and told you to take your cross and go home!"

Black humour serves many social functions. Julie explained, "It helps to build the atmosphere of teamwork, like we are all in this together. It's easier to work with people you laugh with." Jane shared this view saying, "The black humour relieves stress. We laugh so we don't cry. We laugh so we can cry."

### Situational humour

Situational humour may be rooted in the nurse's or patient's actions or discomforts. The bed pan that spills, the water jug that tips over — these situations that could lead to other negative emotions and consequences are turned into positive experiences by finding the humour in the event. One day, as we entered a patient's room with ice water in hand, Jane tripped and flung the water jug into the patient's lap. The patient, who could have become upset, just smiled a crooked smile and said, "Well, at least I'm awake now."

Situational humour humanizes the environment. The nurse and patient involved in such a situation touch each other with humour.

Together they help one another cope with the unexpected. During a conversation Julie said,

> Most of the time it is just the situation. Usually, it is just spontaneous because some things that happen are really funny. Like the other day, one of the doctors wrote an order that said, "Keep trying to get the patient to suck on his balls three times per day." He meant have him use his incentive spirometer machine — but when we read the order, we just totally lost it.

### Divergent humour

Spiegel describes the divergent approach to humour as "arising from disjointed, ill-suited pairing of ideas or situations or presentations of ideas or situations that are divergent from habitual customs."[147] An example of divergent humour is contained in a standing joke in the unit, "Around here, two club sodas equals a party." A field note provides another example of divergent humour.

> A patient's daughter had made multiple trips back and forth in front of the nursing station moving in her Mom's personal belongings. Finally, the daughter said to the nurse I was watching, "That's the last load, just a couple of cases of beer to go." Without hesitation, the nurse replied, "Good, let's put it in the fridge."

Another field note recalls an equally revealing example of divergent humour.

> Coming down the hallway towards us was a tiny elderly lady. Her gait was so unsteady she was at risk for a fall. Maintaining her calm demeanor, the nurse, Julie, approached the woman and taking her securely by the

arm said, "If the police saw you, they would arrest you for impaired driving; let's get you to a wheelchair." They both laughed at the preposterousness of this innocent, angelic grandmother being arrested for anything.

On another occasion, two nurses were discussing possible interventions to assist a very agitated bed-ridden patient. After seriously considering several alternatives without success, Peter lightened the situation by saying, "That man used to be a carpenter — can't we give him a wall to knock down or something?" The image of this very ill man doing something as physical as hospital renovations was very humorous. The laughter stimulated productive discussions focused on solving the problem.

### DEVELOPING THE ATTITUDE

Gelazis contends that nurses have been taught and socialized to maintain a serious demeanor while caring for patients.[148] Humour calls for genuineness and the ability to be yourself, to shed some of this indoctrination.

Hunt claims that humour is a skill and thus can be learned.[149] The nurses in this study agreed that the lighthearted attitude can be developed and practiced. Lana said, "Developing a sense of the humorous begins by learning to laugh at yourself." Jane commented that, "people who can laugh at themselves will always be amused" and Gelazis adds that, "Laughing at oneself has been associated with maturity.... It is a use of oneself as the primary instrument of healing."[150]

Our sense of humour evolves. As Stephen Leacock, the well-known Canadian humourist, observed over half a century ago, "Both the sense of humour and the expression of it undergoes, in the course of history, an upward and continuous process."[151] The nurses were sensitive to this developmental change. Jane explained, "I can see a real change in myself and in my attitude over the years of nursing. Things I laugh about today, I would have cried about a few years ago. Now I can see the fun in things while I see the sadness." This attitude can be built, like a muscle is developed, with exercise.

Benner and Wrubel conclude that humour can "reframe a situation; however, effective use of humor requires a deep background of understanding of the situation and at least a modicum of trust and respect."[152] The nurses I observed had these qualities. They understood from their previous experiences how the patient might be feeling; they had developed trusting relationships with their patients; they were respectful of the uniqueness of each individual and each situation; and they had cultivated in themselves a humorous attitude. Consequently, they were able to use humour appropriately and effectively as a nursing intervention.

Adopting a humorous attitude allows us to reassert our invulnerability and refuse to submit to threat or fear. When we laugh at ourselves, we have a healthy perspective and are able to neutralize our shortcomings. By assuring a humorous attitude, we open ourselves to the world and extend ourselves to others.

### THE TRILOGY REVIEWED

All three of the themes identified — dialogue of silence, mutual touch, and sharing the lighter side of life — share commonalities. Using these approaches involves both the patient and the nurse. Any interpersonal exchanges are experienced by the participants together. Both parties are affected by the action or the attitude. It is not a matter of one doing to the other; it is a shared experience, doing with one another.

Silence, touch, and lightheartedness are avenues of communication. They are means by which the nurses enter their patients' worlds and share their experiences, via messages that are sent and received instantaneously.

Silence, touch, and lightheartedness are all qualities and forces that are felt, that cannot be measured. As Leacock said, "You cannot weigh an argument in a balance, measure social forces with a slide rule, or resolve humour with a stethoscope."[153] I believe this is the case for silence and touch as well.

The complexity and universality of each theme is evident. My synopsis of observations and analyses cannot fully capture the intricacy of the myriad of approaches to patient care. However, it is possible that the stories, poems, and narratives leave us with a greater insight than we had previously.

They all expose a basic honesty. Through touch, silence, and laughter, a part of each person comes into view, no longer hidden from the other. This opening of the spirit of the nurse and patient allows care to be given and care to be received.

—

**THE CAN OPENERS**

Touch, laughter, silence
these are can openers
to your spirit.

They pry off the lid
to your soul
and let me peek inside.

—

# chapter six

## THE EFFECTS OF EXEMPLARY
## NURSING CARE

In chapter 6, I illustrate the results of using the three aspects of exemplary nursing care presented in chapters 3, 4, and 5: touch, silence and lightheartedness.

### CONNECTING

Clayton, Murray, Horner, and Green define connecting as "the transpersonal experiences 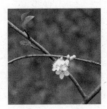 and feelings that lead to the sense of connection, attachment, or bonding between a nurse and a patient."[154] This connection between nurse and patient is a complex and important part of the phenomenon of exceptional nursing practice.

Connecting, as described by the nurses, involves several components: noting the similarities between nurse and patient, recognizing that the patient was once well, and participating in the patient's experience.

—

**STEPPING INTO YOUR WORLD**
There are moments when I feel like
I have stepped inside your world.
For just a flash,
I feel your pain,
I know your despair.
I sense what it's like to have cancer
from the inside looking out
at a world of people who are fit and well.
My God — it's so tragic.
My God — it's so unfair.

—

## Recognizing the similarities

Maureen told me this story about a connection that occurred very naturally with one patient. This connection developed partially out of mutual recognition of their similarities.

A young mother of two kids had a brain tumour. This was a real warm relationship from the beginning. We shared — we were very close. I was overwhelmed sometimes by what she was going through. I remember how grateful I was for her that she had such a supportive husband. I was in awe of how much strength she possessed. Whenever you admire someone, you want to be close to them and study them. She wrote me a poem that I got just after she died. She taught me a lot about me, and made a real difference in my life. I may forget her name, but I will always remember her and the ways she was like me, and the ways I wanted to be like her.

—

**YOU AND ME: THE SYMMETRY**
As different as cold and hot,
soft and hard,
happy and sad,
you and me.
Yet even where differences are vast,
there are similarities.

We do share...
a desire to be needed,
a desire to be loved,
a desire to be acknowledged,
a desire to be remembered.

—

Marie told me this story of a patient she connected with, although on the surface they seemed very different.

She was sixteen years old. I'd been her nurse right from the very first admission day. We'd grown so very close. Unlike me, she was a mother, and now a very sick leukemic — just too much for her 16 years to handle. To me, she was just a young teenage girl in need of her mom.

She returned from a pass one Sunday and eagerly searched me out to give me a photo of her 12 month old baby girl, Amy. I remember how proud she was as she showed me the photo and how carefully she wrote on the back and handed it to me. We both smiled and talked about her little one. I listened intently as a non-mother. This would be the last evening we would spend together in such a happy carefree way.

Years later, after I had my own little girl, I was looking over an old desk calendar. Amy's photo slipped out, and I recalled that evening we had shared. I now knew the joy of being a mom — the pride of having your own child — and I realized that little Amy brought some beautiful rays of sunshine to a young teenage girl's last days.

—

**IN ME, YOU**

We recognize ourselves in others.

In you I see me,
my potential as a mother,
as a woman,
and as someone who will die soon.

The only difference between me and you
is that you are probably closer to your death.

—

This same nurse went on to tell me a story about connecting — finding a common bond — with a patient named Kenny. She said,

I remember Kenny because he called the hospital from his home up north and said he was never coming back to the hospital in the city again. He was a typical teenager — rebelled all the time, didn't do the things he was asked to do; he was non-compliant through and through.

After some coaxing, he did come back to see us for a treatment. I was his nurse. The only thing he really liked was fishing, and I thought, "Bingo — I can relate to fishing." I told him I liked to fish, too, and he said, "You like fishing?" with total disbelief in his voice. I

146

said, "Yah — I can get into it." He tried some lingo on me about hooks and jigs and I passed. Then he said, "I've got something to show you." It was a home video of ice fishing. The whole movie was of a hole in the ice. The odd time he would say, "Did you see that?" Then he would rewind until we both saw the fish. That was our connection. On each visit, I'd always start with, "How was the fishing?"

There is always a connection possible. If it isn't going to be with me, maybe another nurse can do it for that patient.

———

**OVERLAPPING REALITIES**

We are different?
We are the same?
We are essentially the same!

Finding that point where we are the same,
makes caring for each other so natural.

———

*Seeing the former you*

The nurses described the ability to envision patients in their minds as the persons they were before they became ill as an important prerequisite to, and part of, connecting. Three of the exceptional nurses made these comments.

When you see that stretcher coming down the hall with a new admission, the patient at first means very little to you. But as you get to know them, look at pictures of them before they were ill, see their personalities and features reflected in their family members, you feel a lot different about them.

Your first contact with a new patient before you get to know them is hard. They are usually bald, jaundiced, thin — not nice looking. And then you go into their room and start talking to them and all that disappears. You see that person as the person they were before. As you find out more about them, you see the person inside — you see their spirit, their soul. I'm not sure what to call it — maybe their essence. The average person on the street would be repulsed by their appearance, but the people here who care so much see only their beautiful side.

I always try to picture what the patient was like before they got cancer. I ask questions about what they liked and didn't like — about their hobbies, their work, their family interactions. Knowing these things just helps me give better care.

In a sense, "knowing" the pre-illness person facilitates establishing a nurse–patient connection. Maureen commented, "It's just easier somehow to connect with the patient if you have known them since their initial diagnosis or at least if you see pictures of them from before [they got sick]. Then you have the total picture of that patient." She went on to tell me this story.

The patient in room 18 was a sixteen-year-old girl with an astrocytoma. I knew she had been admitted many times before and had become a favorite of the staff, although I had never met her. I knocked on her door and entered the room. There in the bed lay a person; it was hard to know the age, or even the sex, of the body lying there staring at me with wide eyes. Her face was swollen — typical of the cushingoid syndrome that develops with prolonged steroid use. Her hair was sparse and patchy, revealing her scalp. Her facial features drooped and her mouth sagged in one corner. Her body was swollen and her arm movements uncoordinated. There was evidence of anxiety in her eyes as she looked at my unfamiliar face.

I approached her, gently laying my hand on her arm, and said, "My name's Maureen. I will be your nurse tonight." Some incoherent noises came from her mouth as she acknowledged what I was saying. She pointed towards a list with words on it, showing me her name — Maureen. I nodded and said, "I know — your name is Maureen, too. You know, Maureens are the best people. We should have a great time tonight." She grinned and pointed to a picture on her bedstand. The picture was of a beautiful, young woman with long, brown hair and a gorgeous smile. Maureen watched me — waiting for me to make the connection that this picture was of her.

I looked at her and smiled. "Is this a picture of you?" I asked. Tears filled her eyes as she nodded. Then I realized how important it was to her that I knew who she was before she got sick, and that she was still that person. She taught me something that night that I will never forget.

When I asked Maureen about this story she elaborated on the lesson she received that night saying, "I learned that, to provide the very best care, I need to know who that person was before becoming sick and to realize that person and their history is very important to the patient I am now caring for."

Moria gave me the same message when she said, "You have to see past the smells, cachexia, crumpled, broken, misshapen bodies to see the former radiance." One day on the unit when we were caring for a patient who was in such a state, Moria said, "She must have been such a beautiful woman — just look at her skin and her hair."

—

**INSIDE THE PEBBLE**

Every pebble,

no matter how chipped and broken,

potentially contains

a dusting of gold.

—

*Participating in the patient's experience*

When I asked Cindy how she defined a "good day," she said, "I know I have had a good day when I make the connection with a patient, when I feel comfortable sitting on their bed or giving them a hug — when I am part of their experience." Many of the nurses' stories describe times when they made this connection with their patients by participating in their experiences through sharing their pain, suffering, joy, or an intimate moment with them. The following is one of Marie's examples of such an encounter:

> I want to tell you about one of my patients. He was a doctor himself — very ill, very uptight, very much in need of control over his care. I had known him only vaguely in his previous role as a doctor on the unit, and now here he was — my patient. I was called to perform a difficult procedure on him, and I remember thinking, "How can I handle this? How can I make a connection with him?"

> Before I brought in all of my materials for the procedure, I went in and sat down with him. I told him my name and said, "You probably don't remember me, but

I do remember when you were a doctor here." I said that I really remembered him and that he stood out in my mind because he was so personable and that I was impressed by how he had treated the nurses and his patients. I would never have been able to tell him these things except for the situation — at that moment, he was in a more vulnerable position than I was. I just said what I felt — that I was really sorry that he had cancer.

That time together was important. It made both of us feel at ease and I was able to do the procedure then without anxiety. When he came back for another treatment a week later, he asked for me. I was glad I had taken the time to make that personal bond. He talked to me about his plans — the things he could never do that he wanted to do. Even after he knew that he was going on with his disease and he stopped the treatments, he would always stop by and talk to me. I really miss him.

In this example, Marie participated in her patient's experience by spending time with him, sharing "secrets" with him, and giving of herself. All of these are part of sustaining the nurse-patient connection.

Marie shared this example of her participation in another patient's experience.

She was young, sweet, and soft-spoken. I just wanted to mother her. She had been through so much. She didn't really understand what disease she had — let alone that it was bad. We were like mother and daughter from the beginning. That was the nature of our relationship. With her I would just say, "You have to do this...," "Listen to me...," "Come on, you can do it...." I wouldn't use that approach with any other patients but, with her, it just really fit.

I feel as if I shared in her experience. I was with her — at least in mind — from the moment she was admitted until her last day. She was my patient; I was her nurse. When she died, so did a part of me.

—

### THE CONNECTION

An unseen thread joins our spirits.
As we journey through this time together
we share ourselves with one another.
Things that would never be
appropriate to say to even my
closest friend,
are, with you, not only appropriate,
but necessary.

We both know that time is short.
To leave things unsaid now, is to
leave them unsaid forever.

—

## AFFIRMING THE VALUE OF THE PATIENT

The connection between patient and nurse is related to affirming the value of the patient. An underlying focus of the care given by exceptionally competent nurses is an acknowledgment of the patient as an important and worthy individual — as someone who has value. This is a part of the nurses' belief system as they enter into nurse-patient relationships; it is reflected in the nursing care they give, and it is an effect of their nursing actions and interactions.

It appears that there are at least four major means by which nurses communicate to patients that they are valued. Specifically, nurses help patients to be remembered; they help patients to create meaning out of their experiences; they treat patients with respect to help them maintain dignity; and they help patients see their possibilities — to find hope.

### Helping the patients feel they will be remembered

In an interview, Julie said,

> People can take almost anything — but they can't take being forgotten. Anybody, if they have one wish, they want to be remembered. Every person wants to make some significant contribution. Sometimes it is part of my role to help them with this.

—

**REMEMBER ME**

When I am gone,
I have only one request,
remember me.

Say my name,
and remember me.
Touch my things,
and remember me.
Recall my smile,
and remember me.

I simply have to be more than dust.
Dust is just dust,
and when the wind blows it scatters
and is forever
lost.

—

153

Julie wrote this story:

> A young mother of a three-year-old was facing her own death. She had brain mets that were interfering with her cognitive and motor abilities to complete the many handicraft projects she wanted to finish and bequeath to her child. The disease was progressing quickly; she was overcome more and more with fatigue and confusion. She asked me to finish a counted cross-stitch picture for her, but instead we packaged up the partially finished picture — thread and all — with a note that said, "My dear, dear child…When you want to, please finish this picture, and it will be something you can say we did together…My hand will guide you. Love, Mom."

Jane said, "The patients — especially near the end — just want to be assured they will be remembered. No one can bear the thought that after they are gone, they will disappear and not matter anymore." I asked her how she responds to these concerns, and she answered, "Usually, I just help them believe that people will remember them. I say, 'Let's talk about the people who will remember you,' and we talk about specific differences they have made in other people's lives."

Lana said, "Sometimes we have to be part of the group that remembers the patient." She talked about the responsibility she feels to remember certain people — especially those who may not have family members who will recall their memory. The nurses told me about gifts, poems, and letters they or the nursing unit had received "in memory" of specific patients. They felt it was part of their role to carry on these memories. Maureen, in telling me about a patient who had written her a poem that she had received just after the patient died, said, "I may forget her name, but I will always remember her. It is just part of what I do."

Jane commented, "A part of remembering is recognizing the uniqueness of individuals, because, in remembering, we recall what made that person special. There isn't a patient that isn't special in some way."

*Helping the patients find meaning in their experiences*
Marie stated, "Probably the hardest question I am asked is, 'Why me?', and all the patients ask it in their own way, in their own time. What can I say? It's really, really hard." What she was addressing is the role the nurses play in helping their patients create meaning out of their cancer experience.

Frankl writes about the importance of finding meaning in our experiences. He says,

> To live is to suffer, to survive is to find meaning in suffering. If there is a purpose in life at all, there must be a purpose in suffering and dying.... If one succeeds, one will continue to grow in spite of all indignities. He who has a why to live can bear with almost any how.[155]

It seems from the examples provided by the exemplary nurses that they work together with their patients to help them find their whys. Expert nurses work at helping patients find meaning, or more precisely, they help their patients make sense out of what is happening to them. In a similar vein Burke commented, "Each person strives to create meaning out of his existence in the world and attempts to gain freedom from crippling fear, anxiety, and guilt."[156]

Some nurses suggested that, when confronted with the possibility of death, the urgency of this search is accelerated. Simultaneously, due to the devastating nature of the disease, this quest becomes more difficult. As Lana said, "How can a person be expected to find meaning in suffering and death? How much more difficult can it get?"

Although the nurses acknowledge that it is a difficult task, they recognize their role in helping the patients with their search for meaning within the limits of their individual circumstances. Julie told me this story of a man she helped to find meaning in a life that had been devastated by more than cancer.

> He was a tall, good-looking man. At his request, there was a "No Visitors" sign on his door. He drew pictures; he discussed world politics. He didn't cry — he didn't laugh; he watched. He gave single word answers. His patient history report said he was an atheist. He had attempted suicide because he did not wish to put his wife through the excruciating process of slowly watching him die. He was admitted to prevent any subsequent suicide attempts.

> I personally believe that, given enough opportunities, even the hardest rock can be — if not cracked — at least warmed by the sun. Initially, that rock was all I saw, but this man taught me about the "sands of time" and the importance of approaching every situation with caring and honesty — and to never judge.

> I am good at making people feel comfortable. I enjoy helping them get rid of a lot of emotional garbage. I knew he needed to have his inner fears affirmed — to come to terms with the grief and the multitude of losses he was encountering. He needed, at least, to search for answers to the question, "Why?" I recognized his lone-liness and his fear. How was I going to let him know I was there to help?

> The opportunity finally arrived one evening. He all of

a sudden said, "Do you believe in God?" I answered carefully, not wanting to shut the doors. I said, "I really don't know about God *per se*. But I do believe in angels."

Regardless of my attempt, his part of the conversation quickly changed to the practical matters at hand — like the size of his pajamas. However, with the passing weeks, we did discuss angels, a little bit about God, grief, anger, hate, and how unfair this was.

He told me a lot about his life. He had been a young family man during the war — an army officer. One day he and his wife went for groceries, leaving their two boys at home. While they were gone, their home was bombed. Their home and family were destroyed. As postwar refugees to Canada, his wife bore another son who died shortly after birth. In an attempt to gather some semblance of normality after all this heartache, they adopted an infant. This child was now in his mid-thirties and mentally handicapped.

I think of him often. I was fortunate to be with him in his last moments. I held his hand. All I could do was stand there and hope that he was seeing his kids. I prayed, "Please, if there is a God, this man deserves to see his kids."

I don't know if it was just the effects of his drugs or what, but when I said to him as he was dying, "Your sons are there," he squeezed my hand. He really did. He squeezed my hand and died. And I sobbed.

—

**FINDING MEANING: THE FIRST STEP**
You listened to me with openness.
Into your willing heart I poured
my fears, my sadness, my guilt.
Now that I am free of these chains
there is a chance I may find serenity.

—

Just by listening to this patient and helping him to relive his stories, Julie set him on the way to being able to find meaning in his experience. Without this opportunity to free oneself of the guilt and pain of past failures and sorrows, it would be difficult for any patient to think clearly about what part the cancer experience plays in his or her life. As Levine said, "When the mind is clear, we can see all the way to the heart" and "when the heart is exposed there are no obstacles in the mind."[157]

Once the "emotional baggage" has been addressed, the nurses talked about the important role of a spiritual element in helping their patients create meaning. As Jane said, "Even if you have never really believed in God or some higher power, it crosses your mind when you face your own — or someone else's — mortality."

Most of the exemplary nurses described their own well-developed spiritual beliefs. Having faith in the existence and mercy of a higher being was important in their ability to help patients create meaning. For example, Julie told me,

> If patients are really struggling with the "Why me?" and "What will happen to me?" questions and they have no faith of their own, I let them cling on to mine until they can find their own. Some of them never do, but I am glad I can help them in this way. I couldn't if I wasn't sure myself — if I hadn't already found my own way.

Marie said that the patients often found meaning in their disease by first considering it part of their destiny, "God's plan for them." As Lana commented, "Once they accept it, they can start to see the glimmer of good in the devastation around their worlds." Jane said, "Acceptance of their situation lets them get back control so they can make sense of the chaos and disruption the illness can cause."

—

**SOARING TO NEW HEIGHTS**
Past the bottom there is an end,
your wings will find their strength once more,
flight again will be your friend,
and onward, upward, you shall soar!

—

*Treating patients with respect and helping them maintain dignity*

Treating their patients with respect and helping them maintain dignity was another way these exceptional nurses showed their patients they were valued. The respect they have for their patients prompted their concern for maintenance of patient dignity. In many of the stories told, this concern underlay the nurses' choices and actions. Frequently, the nurses were patient advocates in an attempt to provide the patients with quality of life as they defined it. As the following story illustrates, doing so can foster patient dignity.

He was only nineteen years old — far, far away from home and desperately in need of a bone marrow transplant. His home was in a small Native community in northern Canada. He was Native, and this was his first trip outside the area in which he lived. Naturally, I expected that my task would be to support him and prepare him for his trip to Toronto for his transplant. But the more time I spent with Ralph, the more I realized he did not share those plans and hopes. Ralph always amazed me because he was insightful, spiritual, and truly at peace with his situation. He was also very alone, frightened, and intimidated by the hospital surroundings. A bone marrow transplant would mean more loneliness and a greater separation from his family and home. A transplant at this stage of his lengthy illness provided only limited hope for a prolongation of life.

Ralph confided in me that his only desire was to return home to be with his family, to experience a familiar sunset before he died. I knew in my heart this could be the only choice for him...Ralph was an inspiration to me. His decision was not popular with his physician who was disturbed by his "giving up," but Ralph never gave up on his decision.

I, along with my colleagues, were resolved that going home was the only correct plan for Ralph. We presented Ralph's position to the doctors, and defended it adamantly. The bone marrow transplant was cancelled.

Ralph never did return home, but died in room 72 surrounded by his mother, brothers, and sisters. He was at peace, and so was I. I truly missed him for some time after. The medical goals of cure and treatment may often be less important when we can clearly distinguish between quality and quantity of life.

———

**LINKING RESPECT AND DIGNITY**
Your body,
your right
to decide
its future.

My role,
to respect that right
and help you
maintain your dignity.

———

Patient dignity was also maintained through nursing actions that helped patients know that they were still important, that their lives still mattered. The following is an excerpt from a letter I wrote to one of the exceptional nurses documenting my observation of her in such a situation.

Dear Moria:
Today I watched in reverence as you cared for your patient. So gently you removed the mountain of bandages that covered what once was his back and buttocks. You respected his privacy by placing a tiny towel over his chest — the only part of his body that didn't need to be exposed during the procedure. I was moved by this symbolic gesture. You respected him; he was more than a patient to you — he was someone you cared about. The smells when you removed the dressings were so bad. I wanted to turn away, but you showed no sign that it bothered you at all. In fact, you moved closer — carrying on a cheerful conversation with him about his life, his work, his grandchildren. In doing these things, you maintained the dignity of a man who probably had only a thread of it left.

—

**PRIVACY IN A VERY PUBLIC SPACE**
Masterful creation
of the illusion of privacy
does wonders to protect the
last remaining grains
of pride and self-respect.

—

Often times, it was just the respectful ways that the nurses carried out their nursing tasks which communicated to the patients that they were important. The following field notes documented some of the little things the nurses did for the patients that I believe helped the patients to feel valued.

She takes an infinite amount of time with each patient. Mrs. Long asked to have her legs elevated. Moria makes minute adjustments to her leg positions until the patient indicates that the angle and the supporting pillows are perfectly positioned. Even after the sign of approval by the patient, Moria waits to make sure everything is satisfactory.

The attention to detail is remarkable. Warming the towels in the drier so they are cozy after a bath, warming the lotion in the microwave, warming the milk at bed time — all of these take time, but the actions seem to help the patients feel important, valued, more worthy. No request is too much for these nurses. In fact, the patients seldom need to ask. The nurses anticipate needs the patients don't even know they have. The patient is ringing her bell every few minutes. When the nurse I am watching answers her call, the patient's complaint is that she can't find her bell. Later she rings again to tell the nurse she doesn't want to be disturbed. Each time, the nurse answers the summons with sincere interest and pleasant patience.

Peter said to me, "Helping patients to feel important can be as simple as knocking on their doors before entering their rooms or asking them what time they would like their baths." Marie concluded,

Making the patient feel like they are the most important person in the world, even if it is just for the moments you are with them, that should be our goal — that has been my goal. Patients are the priority. It's the little things that make a patient feel important, like the way you enter a room. I consciously slow down my pace as I enter. I take time to sit down in the patient's room and really listen to their concerns. I attend to their needs in short order, not waiting to be reminded. If possible, I anticipate their needs before they ask — like offering them an extra pillow or dealing with a red skin area. You just let them know that they still matter. Even if it is just for this moment, you matter.

The nurses I observed continued to show respect and maintain the dignity of their patients — even after they were deceased. In a field note I wrote,

As we enter the dead woman's room, the nurse dims the lights, and tiptoes across the floor to draw the curtains. She talks softly to the woman as she prepares her body for the morgue. In a very quiet voice, she bids the woman, her patient, goodbye.

The importance of showing respect and maintaining patient dignity is supported by Benner. She writes, "Almost no intervention will work if the nurse-patient relationship is not based on respect."[158]

### Helping the patients find and maintain hope

By helping the patients find and maintain hope, the nurses caused the patients to feel they still mattered. The following untitled, anonymous poem, posted on the wall of the nursing unit where this study took place, is a concrete symbol of the importance of maintaining hope.

—

Cancer is so limited....
It cannot cripple love,
corrode faith,
eat away peace,
destroy confidence,
kill friendship,
shut out memories,
silence courage,
invade the soul,
quench the spirit.
The greatest enemy is not the disease,
but despair.

—

After reading this poem, Jane said, "If the patients see no hope — no possibilities for even their immediate future — they are left with despair. But it is part of my goal to help them see possibilities, and set goals that are attainable."

Julie described some of the ways she helps patients realize and accept their limited potential without taking away their hope. She said,

First, you have to honest with patients. People can take a "yes" or a "no" very easily as long as you are being straight with them. When someone is lying there dying, nauseated, and in pain, the last thing they want to hear is, "It's going to be okay." At that moment, it is not going to be okay, and that moment is a year long. Cut the crap.

If they say, "Am I dying?", you say, "Yes, you are dying." They are so content with that because someone is telling them the truth. You say to them, "I'm not going to lie to you." Lying to patients destroys their hope. It lets them down. If you lie to them and tell them they will be able to do something and then they can't, they won't chance hoping again.

If they say to you, "Will I be able to walk?" and they won't, say, "No — but let's try sitting up in a chair." If they ask you, "Can I go home again?" and they can't, say, "Probably not but let's try a pass for two hours or maybe you can just get out of your room." Just give them something. We don't have the right to destroy their hope. I never promise my patients something I can't deliver.

———

**SEEING POTENTIAL**

Your body has been cruel to you,

harnessing you,

limiting your possibilities.

I am here to free your shackles

and set your spirit soaring,

just by helping you see your choices.

———

Hope is a belief that something good lies ahead. It is not denying reality. Realistic hope can help the dying person face reality, while it also gives strength to go on living. Jane said, "I think giving patients hope is important. I used to think that being cheerful was a way of giving hope, but now I know it is helping them find courage."

—

**INFECTIOUS HOPE**

Hope.

It cannot be taught,

or bought,

but can it be caught?

—

In this story, Maureen described how she used her nursing skills to help her patient maintain hope.

This patient was in a lot of pain. We had given her breakthrough medication, but it didn't work and she was crying out. The nurse who was assigned to her was upset and didn't know what to do. She asked me for help, so I went into the room and calmly said, "We are going to try something different." I didn't have a plan when I walked in or even when I said we were going to try something different; I just knew we had to give her some hope.

First, I tried visualization — a Hawaiian beach; that didn't work. So I went into muscle relaxation and, sure enough, it worked — probably because the analgesic had kicked in by then, too. But the distractions of trying these alternatives kept her mind off her pain and let her know we were not going to give up on controlling her pain.

---

**HOPE IS TO LIFE**

Hope.
Without it what is life?
Bleak,
onerous,
hopeless?

Hope.
With it what is life?
Lively,
promising,
possible?

---

In commenting about hope, Lana said,

It is probably the greatest need our patients have. Those without hope just give up and lead a poor quality of life. Those with hope have power over their disease and live a good life until they die. The only problem is, hope is difficult or maybe impossible to dispense because it is a quality of the spirit.

One of my field notes reads,

It seems strange to write about death and hope in the same sentence, but where would the dying be without hope? Those who can't find it collapse inwardly and die before they are dead. Those who somehow discover or choose hope have the elusive quality of life the nurses I'm watching desire for their patients.

On the importance of hope for the dying patient, McHutchion writes,

The hope for the miracle of cure becomes hope for a miracle of care. Patients and families believe that when pain and symptoms of the disease and side effects from treatments and medications are controlled, the patient and family caregiver are freed to live toward a good death.[159]

In another journal entry, I recorded an encounter where a dying man was helped to find the strength to continue hoping for the miracle of care.

A physician approached the nurse I was watching and asked her to come take a look at Mr. Bill Selsby. Entering the room, we find a man lying in bed — silent, and staring at the wall, his eyes fixed. The doctor concludes that the patient is close to death and that the diagnostic test scheduled for Mr. Selsby that day should be cancelled.

After the physician leaves, the nurse does her own assessment of the patient. She goes close to him and studies him very intensely. Placing her hand on his forehead she says, "Bill, are you sad? Are you sad because today is your birthday?" She stays in this pose for a few minutes — waiting for a response, a signal, a clue from the patient. I see nothing. She sees what she needs to see.

Leaving the room, the nurse walks up to the doctor and says, "I think you are wrong about Mr. Selsby — his eyes are reacting. He is not dying; he is just down and depressed."

During the day as we visit Bill's room, he becomes more and more responsive. The nurse talks to him about his life — asking him questions about his children and his birthday wishes. At first he doesn't say much, but eventually he begins to talk.

Just before change of shift, the nurse gathers her colleagues together to help her surprise Bill with a cake. Together they sing the most rousing and sincere happy birthday song I have ever heard. The man who was supposedly taking his last breath cuts the cake and eats a piece with his tea, which the nurse had carefully steeped to his liking and served to him in a china cup.

In a final demonstration of caring, she places a birthday kiss on Bill's forehead — setting an example for the other nurses, who follow her lead. As we leave the room and bid Bill a happy evening, I see the sparkle of life that has returned to those eyes. Bill has hope.

—

**HAPPY BIRTHDAY**

"Happy birthday to you.
Happy birthday to you."
You sing with enthusiasm.
You sing with warmth.
You sing in unison.

In the lines
between your words
you sing this message...
Bill, you may not have many
more birthdays,
but let's just celebrate
this incredibly important birthday moment,
and the hope that it brings.

—

## AFFIRMING THE VALUE OF THE NURSE

As the patient is affirmed by the nurse's actions and their interactions, the nurse is also affirmed. From the observations and the comments of the nurses, this seems to happen in two major ways. First, the nurses come to know that they are making a difference in the lives of their patients or their patients' families. Second, like the patients, the nurses also find meaning in their experiences.

Human beings need to feel they are important. One way that they do this is by helping or adding happiness to other human beings. The exemplary nurses often commented that they found their work rewarding — in part because, through their work, they were able to make a difference in the lives of others. When asked to elaborate on their feelings about their work, participating nurses made the following comments:

> A lot of nursing is doing for others. When I do something for my patient and it is successful, I feel valued — like what I do is constructive, and I am worthy. It's a great feeling.

> I just know that almost every day when I come to work I am going to change somebody's life. It's an awesome power. I take it really seriously. These people with cancer, they are so vulnerable, so needy. I am privileged to be part of their lives at this time when they need me so much. I always feel needed by my patients — and when I can meet their needs, it really makes me happy.

> The most rewarding thing for me is taking patients from situations where they are in a lot of distress, or confused and cognitively impaired, and doing a few simple measures that help them to be alert so they can talk to their

families and be comfortable...It is so satisfying to give them some quality back to their lives.

The rewards are the little things — seeing individuals come back when they have been through a long journey and seeing them triumph. It's a real joy to share that with them. Even if the patient has died, to have the family members come to you and greet you like you were a real special part of their lives is a great feeling. I think of few careers where you can interact with people so closely and feel so helpful to someone, and I feel I really make a difference. It is important to me that what I do is worthwhile.

—

**TO BE VALUED**
I am so alone,
my companions likewise.

But, if I can be vital to but one other,
even for a moment,
I increase my own happiness
by at least one hundred fold.

—

Maureen told me a story about making a difference in a family's life. She said,

This is a story about a young couple. He was diagnosed with colon cancer, and he was only 32 years old. He had two children and so did I. He was really withdrawn all the time and the only thing that could get to him was humour, so I used to joke with him and that would get him talking a little. He was in excruciating pain, but he didn't stop doing the things he loved — like driving his tractor. His wife and I really hit it off; we had a lot in common. She would call me about his pain and other things. One day she called. He was really in trouble, so we asked her to bring him to the hospital.

When he got here, I could see he was near death. He was confused, dehydrated, atrophied. I took his wife aside and talked with her. I told her exactly what I was seeing. I said that I noticed a big change in him since the last time I saw him. I didn't have to tell her that he was dying; she already knew. She told me that it was important to him to die at home, so I set about arranging things, medications, home care — all the things they needed to make it possible, and we sent them home. He died the next day.

It was an extraordinary time for me because I really felt like I made a difference in their lives. They were important to me — not because they taught me a whole lot, but because they made a difference in my life, too.

Julie wrote a story about feeling like she made a difference in a patient's life with a very small, but authentic, gesture of caring.

There's the time I was "out for coffee" (I don't even drink coffee) with the wife of a former patient. Meeting me again was difficult for her as I represented a very sad time in her life. I had shared the approach to, and death of, her husband. They had obviously shared a special, loving relationship. She wanted to talk with me again, but it was not without a flood of memories. While we drank our coffee, she described to me a moment that the three of us had shared, to which she had often returned during her bereavement. This is the moment.

One time on my perpetual medication rounds, I entered her husband's room. I found her and her husband both asleep. He was lying on his bed. She had her head on his chest, and he had his fingers interlaced in her hair. It was a peaceful and loving sight. I could not interrupt, so I simply wrote them a note on the first scrap of paper I could find — a little, yellow sticky. The note said, "Was here — please call when you're awake. You looked so peaceful, just couldn't interrupt. Your Med. Nurse."

Much to my surprise, she had kept the note. She pulled it from her purse that day. It was dog-eared and tattered, but she still had it! Her husband had a huge funeral. There were probably hundreds of Hallmark cards. It had been more than a year ago. She had travelled, she was doing well, but she had saved this little seemingly insignificant yellow sticky note. It was a reminder to me that, yes, we all may secretly wish for fame and fortune — the big things are so obvious — but it's the little things that really do make a difference. My little thing had made a big difference to her. I felt so good.

When I asked about the most satisfying aspect of her job, Marie told me this story.

Last week, a patient's wife came in and wanted to talk to me about her husband's passing. Weeks earlier when I was his nurse, I felt like I was one of her family, and it was a really rewarding time though there were a lot of difficult moments. Now, after his death, she was reaching out to me again. There were many people she could have chosen to reach out to, including family members, but she chose me.

The display of thank-you cards on the nursing unit is another concrete acknowledgement of the difference the nurses make in patients' lives. During visits to their homes, some of the nurses showed me personal cards, tokens, letters, and poems they had received from their patients. These were prized symbols of the difference they had made in the lives of others — stored over the years, kept with a sense of sacredness. The following are excerpts from these messages sent to the exceptionally competent nurses.

My grandmother's life ended with dignity and self-respect. By giving this gift to her, not only was her death respectable, but her life (to the end) was surrounded with love.

What comfort and peace you brought to my Mother. I will never forget you.

Once in a while you meet someone who is really special. You are my special angel.

As I think back over all that we have been through together, I realize that I couldn't have done it without you. I am eternally grateful.

—

**THE MIRACLE CIRCLE**
Sometimes,
when I think about
the vastness and complexity of the world,
I am overwhelmed.
I feel so unimportant,
so insignificant.

Then,
I meet you,
and with a small gesture, lovingly given,
I make you feel valued.

The result is a miracle,
when you feel important,
so do I.
It's so simple.
It's so profound.

—

*Finding meaning in the experience*
As the nurses found meaning in their own experiences with caring
for cancer patients, they came to feel valued. Like the patients, the
nurses struggled to find this meaning. Making a positive difference
in the lives of their patients and the patients' families is one of the
ways the nurses found meaning. However, they did tell me of other
ways this meaning was realized.

Exceptional nurses value continued personal and professional
learning. They seek challenges that facilitate this goal, and their
work provides these challenges. For many of the nurses, having this
opportunity for ongoing enhancement was a part of finding meaning
in their work. As Jane said, "Everyday, I learn something new about
cancer, or about caring, or about me." This finding was reflected in
other comments.

When I first started here, I planned to stay maybe a year — but now it is two years later, and I am still here. When I ask myself why, I realize it is because I still have a lot to learn here.

I just can't imagine a job where you know it all — where you could do everything perfectly all the time. This work is so demanding, so challenging, so dynamic that knowing it all would never happen. That's good. That's the way I like it. That's why I stay.

I really enjoy the opportunity to continue to learn. I go to cancer conferences and come back inspired, proud of what I do, and full of new ideas. I read journals and I'm happy to have the chance to try out the new ideas with my patients.

We can still keep on learning. Even if you have learned the lesson once, you still have to be reminded from time to time. That's the beauty of this job. You never, never stop [learning].

—

**CHALLENGE SEEKERS**
You only become greater
if you are first confronted with
not knowing how.

In your wisdom you recognize this,
and seek
and welcome
the obstacle of challenge.

—

The exceptional nurses recognized that they were not perfect nurses or perfect people — that they were not finished their journeys. They suggested that they did not ever expect that they would achieve perfection, although they enjoyed working toward that unattainable possibility. The result was a yearning for continued learning and growth. In a letter to Peter I wrote,

> I am impressed with your interest in continuing to learn, developing your nursing abilities along with your personal qualities and philosophies. One important point that you helped me to bring to light is that exceptionally competent nurses are not perfect. I think most people equate exceptional with infallible, but that isn't true for any of the nurses I observed. What is true is that exceptional nurses are self-aware, they know their own limitations and their strengths and they adjust their practice accordingly. In addition, they have a desire for life-long learning. I believe this may demonstrate a level of maturity that only rare people reach.

Beyond seeking and overcoming challenges, there were other ways that the nurses I studied found meaning in their experience. For example, Jane described how helping the patients create meaning from their experiences actually helped her create meaning from her experience. She said,

> Working here, I have come to grips with a lot of the heavy issues — you know, life, death, religion, love, family. You have to help the patients with these issues first, but when you do, you can't help also working through the same issues in your own life. It just happens sort of naturally.

As we discussed it further, she began to debate in her mind which comes first. She said,

> I'm not sure if you deal with your own issues first to prepare you to help your patients, or if being confronted with their issues forces you to quickly determine what life is all about. Maybe you go back and forth; you do a little work on your own, and then you help your patients, and then it's back to you. Yes, I think that's it — I work on it with the patients. Confronting their issues with them forces me to face my own circumstances.

In addition, many of the nurses suggested that they found it necessary to find meaning in their lives outside of work in order to find meaning in their work. Again, this was a simultaneous process — working on discovering meaning in all parts of their lives at the same time. However, the agreement was that they found the searches mutually supportive.

---

**FOG LIFTED**

What a vague idea,
the search for meaning.
Yet, once found,
it becomes crystal clear.

---

## JOINT TRANSCENDENCE: LIVING THE EXTRAORDINARY

In writing about transcendence, O'Banion and O'Connell suggest, "Transcendence changes things, the past, the present, and the future. Once transcendence occurs there is no retreating. It is more than the ordinary."[160] Watson is more specific in her description of transcendence, placing her discussion within the context of the nurse-patient relationship. She says,

When both care provider and care receiver are co-participants in caring, the release can potentiate self-healing and harmony in both. The release can allow the one who is cared for to be the one who cares, through the reflection of the human condition that in turn nourishes the humanness of the care provider. In such connectedness they are both capable of transcending self, time and space. Neither stands above the other.[161]

In an earlier work, Watson writes about "transpersonal caring," a situation in which "both the nurse and patient are changed by the actual caring event."[162] She describes this situation as having a "field of its own that is greater than the occasion itself and which allows for the presence of the spirit."[163] To expand further, Watson suggests that when both the patient and the nurse are fully present in the moment there is a feeling of union with the other. In her words, "the event expands the limits of openness and has the ability to expand human capacities."[164]

In some ways, all of the narratives and observations described in this book illustrate a part of this effect of exceptional nursing practice I have called joint transcendence, or what Watson describes as transpersonal caring.[165] Yet, no one story or observed moment illustrates it completely. O'Banion and O'Connell describe the difficulty encountered when one attempts to write about transcendence. They conclude that transcendence "is an experience so far beyond the ordinary...how can we speak of it in everyday words? Of course we cannot."[166]

In following their advice, I have decided to use few words to describe this core concept. Instead, the poem "Shared Journey" attempts to distill from the collection of stories and observations what is meant by joint transcendence.

—

**SHARED JOURNEY**
Together,
nurse and patient
rise above the pain,
suffering,
and despair
of cancer,
and climb to the top of the mountain that
has no summit.

They take turns
carrying one another.
For they know that neither
can make it alone.

In their time together,
they share through touch,
silence,
and lightheartedness.

In their time together,
they learn about themselves,
their needs,
their strengths,
their limitations.
But most important of all
they learn about their similarities.

They both share the common fate
of mortality,
an understanding which makes
the pleasures of life more intense.

They both possess the potential

for knowing joy,

awe,

and wonder.

They both can understand

that though the physical body

may be diseased,

disfigured,

distasteful,

the spiritual body can be healthy,

beautiful,

and whole.

Through the intimacy of their

relationship they discover

they are valued,

they are worthwhile,

that they can,

and do,

make a difference.

Each, in their own way,

creates meaning out of their experience.

As they reach

higher and higher planes

the patient may leave

to take up challenges elsewhere,

while the nurse,

having gained strength

from the journey

is able to carry on.

—

# *chapter seven*

## LESSONS LEARNED

The insights discussed in this final chapter provide both a summary of the themes described and a reservoir of unanswered questions. These understandings and queries represent a refocusing away from the more detailed analysis to a wide-angle view of the practice of exemplary nurses. The insights are divided into two groups: those that have potential significance for nurses, and those of possible interest to other human-services professionals.

### WHAT NURSES SHOULD KNOW

Exemplary nursing practice is not only more complex than I imagined, it is also more 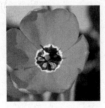 difficult to capture and communicate than I first thought. However, I did gain some important insights about exemplary nurses and some unexpected supplementary insights were revealed circuitously. The following sections include insights arising from the study that may have significance for nurse administrators, researchers, educators, and clinicians.

## Beyond competent care

Exceptional nursing practice is more than competent performance of procedures, although these exemplary nurses were skilled practitioners as well. Though the nurses I studied performed the same procedures as other nurses, their care seemed superior. They changed dressings, administered medications, bathed and positioned patients, assessed vital signs, and served meals as most nurses do — yet the positive effects on them and on their patients were notable. What was it that made their performance of these procedures different?

I suggest that part of the difference between competence and exceptional competence results from the beliefs and values that underlay the nurses' actions. As Wiedenbach says, a nurse's philosophy regarding the significance of life and the worth of each individual determines the quality of nursing care given.[167]

—

**COMPETENT VERSES EXEMPLARY**

I bathe my patient with water.
You bathe your patient in warmth.
I feed my patient toast and porridge.
You feed your patient hope.


I deliver to my patients
medications that make them well.
You deliver to your patients
elixirs that make them whole.

—

## Philosophy: A blueprint for action

The exemplary nurses' beliefs were like a blueprint for action. Their philosophies of nursing practice gave them direction, and because they held firmly to their beliefs, their philosophies gave them strength to go against the system and act as advocates for their patients when necessary.

Marie's story from an earlier chapter about her patient, Ralph, plainly illustrates an association between a nurse's strength of belief and her ability to act as an effective patient ally.

He was only nineteen years old — far, far away from home and desperately in need of a bone marrow transplant. His home was in a small community in northern Canada. He was Native, and this was his first trip outside the area in which he lived. Naturally, I expected that my task would be to support him and prepare him for his trip to Toronto for his transplant. But the more time I spent with Ralph, the more I realized he did not share those plans and hopes. Ralph always amazed me because he was insightful, spiritual, and truly at peace with his situation. He was also very alone, frightened, and intimidated by the hospital surroundings. A bone marrow transplant would mean more loneliness and a greater separation from his family and home. A transplant at this stage of his lengthy illness provided only limited hope for a prolongation of life.

Ralph confided in me that his only desire was to return home to be with his family, to experience a familiar sunset before he died. I knew in my heart this could be the only choice for him. Ralph was an inspiration to me. His decision was not popular with his physician who was disturbed by his "giving up," but Ralph never gave up on his decision.

I, along with my colleagues, were resolved that going

home was the only choice for Ralph. We presented Ralph's position to the doctors and defended it adamantly. The bone marrow transplant was cancelled.

Ralph never did return home, but died in room 72 surrounded by his mother, brothers, and sisters. He was at peace, and so was I. I truly missed him for some time after. The medical goals of cure and treatment may often be less important when we can clearly distinguish between quality and quantity of life.

The most consistent aspects of the philosophies of the exceptional nurses were a belief that life is precious; a respect for the dignity, worth, autonomy, and individuality of each human being; an awareness of the value of self-understanding; a commitment to helping each patient attain the highest quality of life possible, with quality being defined by the patient; an acceptance that death is a natural part of life; and a resolve to act according to their philosophies.

Most importantly, their patients were their reasons for being nurses. As these nurses considered each nursing action or interaction, they thought about how it would affect the quality of life for that particular patient as that patient defined quality. The belief that the patient is the primary consideration seemed to sustain them in their practice. This stance made it easier for the nurses to make decisions and helped them be more confident in upholding those choices.

The nurses would often ask themselves, or their colleagues, "Is this action in this patient's best interest?" before proceeding with an intervention. For example, a patient being cared for by a nurse I was observing seemed close to death. The patient had been prescribed a laxative pill. This nurse was about to administer the drug when she said to me, "I've decided to withhold the medication. I don't want her last memories to be struggling to swallow this."

There were many examples of the exceptional nurses consciously weighing the patient's needs against the directives of the system. For the nurses, their choices became straightforward when their philosophies of nursing were clear.

Yet, the beliefs held by these nurses were not necessarily static. The core ones perhaps were, but generally the nurses' philosophies were being refined over time through their experiences. At any moment, the nurses knew what they believed about each aspect of their practice — yet they were open to changing their beliefs as they encountered new experiences.

—

**MAKING CHOICES**

When you know

what you believe,

choices are no longer

agonizing decisions,

they are readily prescribed

by your beliefs.

—

*The importance of self-awareness*

There were some insights revealed regarding self-awareness, both the role it plays in being or becoming an exceptional practitioner, and how it is developed. It appears the nurses learned most about themselves from others, including colleagues and patients. These people were a mirror in which they recognized themselves. Through their interactions with others, they identified their own limitations; they recognized that no one, including themselves, is perfect and that interdependence leads to the greatest potential for success. In these ways, they discovered both their own uniquenesses and their essential sameness.

In the oncology environment, and possibly in other stressful, urgent contexts, there is potential for developing high levels of self-awareness. Self-awareness was achieved, at least in part, when the nurses turned inward and faced their own existential questions. The oncology environment may be a catalyst for such introspection.

It appears that, because the exemplary nurses knew themselves, they were prepared to confront the issue of their own mortality, to understand the meaning of death — theirs and others. For them, being prepared to die was to understand what it would mean to cease to exist as the selves they are. The nurse who understands this may be better prepared to give exceptional care to seriously ill people. Introspection and experience seemed to be ways by which the nurses developed this self-awareness.

The exemplary nurses understood why they were nurses. They believed that they had chosen to be nurses, and they deliberately and regularly reconfirmed this choice. They also chose to enjoy their work and to learn from it.

The nurses' actions and behaviours stemmed in part from an intense knowledge of self and acceptance of self. Self-awareness meant knowing what they believed about nursing, but it also included knowing their own physical, emotional, and spiritual selves, plus understanding their own limitations.

## The physical self

The physical self includes knowing one's body and ensuring physical needs for sleep, exercise, and nutrition are met. In talking about striving for "total wellness," Julie said,

> I take care of myself.... If you are frustrated trying to meet your own needs, how the wonder are you going to meet someone else's needs? If you haven't decided what is important for yourself and what isn't important, how are you going to take these fragile family situations and give them any direction or help?

She went on to describe the part her uniform and her physical appearance play in her success as a nurse.

> You don't have to wear a label that says you are a nurse when you wear a uniform. I stretch the limit of the uniform. I have always been a provocative dresser. I do it as a statement of individuality, because I like to be identified. If you care enough about yourself to dress well and appropriately, then the patients will feel cared about, too. If you go looking like a slob, how can they possibly have confidence in you? If you can't care enough to put your best foot forward, then how can you care about your patients? If you can't have your sweater matching your uniform, then you don't care very much...and the more you care about yourself, then the more you are available to care about others.

## The spiritual self

Most of the nurses provided insights into their beliefs about the spiritual self. In several cases, this sense of self developed as they cared for dying patients, or faced questions about the existence of a greater power, life, and death. Some talked about their belief in God, a higher power, or angels, and the power of praying for and with their patients. The following story illustrates this well.

> The process of dying can take a long, long time. Mr. Paul had been in the last stages for about two weeks. He was a very religious and devout family man. We had shared many memories together, many discussions in the previous months of his illness. I was there when he was initially diagnosed and had come to know his children quite well. His family had been keeping vigil day and night at his bedside. They had been reading to

him, praying his very favorite prayers, and leaving him distance as well. He was very at peace with his dying. But, why, why was this taking so long?

It was Tuesday morning. I was not his nurse that day. His nurse met me in the hallway. She felt that soon he would die. His apnea spells were far too long, his extremities cold and mottled. I whisked through the hallway and caught sight of his wife and two daughters. I clutched one hand and one shoulder and whispered, "It's time." I'm not sure if they knew at that time what I was suggesting. I walked them into the room as quickly as possible. I placed one of his hands in his wife's, and the other hand in his daughter's. I nodded and simply stated, "He's going home." Tears flowed as they said goodbye. I cried too. No matter how prepared you are for death, the final moments are always hard. I felt very privileged to be present during this time as many of his family were not there yet. His other children had all been called by this time, and they were on their way.

In a short while, all of his children and their respective families arrived, and we ushered them into the room. They formed a circle around him, joined hands, and extended their hands to me, inviting me into their family. Together they prayed for his safe journey.

I can't tell you how very special I felt to be a part of that intimate circle. It was a gift that would give me a great deal of strength in the deaths I would stand by in the days to come.

Another story speaks about the power of prayer in Marie's practice.

She was exactly my age. But that's where our similarities ended. She arrived back early from a Sunday pass, and we were overlooking the city from the window of her hospital room. It was a hot summer afternoon. She was worried about her only family member, her ten-year-old son. He was so precious, and I had come to care for him deeply. I recall he was wise — far, far beyond his years — and had taken over as caregiver for his Mom.

His Mom had advanced breast cancer, which was extremely rare for someone her age. She had suffered greatly all her youth in a war-torn country. Recently, she had escaped to Canada and here had suffered an abusive marriage. This all preceded her fatal diagnosis. She was very much alone. As I learned more and more about her, I was chilled by her history. As we talked that day, tears streamed from her eyes. She turned to me and asked, "Why, Marie? Why do these things happen? Does no one care about us?"

We were watching people outside enjoying the summer day. I immediately felt trapped inside as she did. Nothing I had been taught made sense right now. I could not answer her. Tears clouded my eyes as my gaze met hers; all I could say was, "I don't know why. I wish I could tell you."

I thought, "What a feeble, feeble answer." I paused for a long time sitting with her. Then I opened up and told her that I was a Christian and that the only thing I knew to offer her were my prayers. I exposed myself to a patient like I had never done before. She thanked me and then said, "I am a Buddhist; can I pray for you too?" I said I would be grateful to receive her prayers.

Perhaps there is something more we had in common. We both had a good Sunday evening.

Marie added a postscript during a follow-up conversation. She said, "I was just totally blown away that someone could have such a devastating life. I didn't know how to answer her, so all I could do was pray for her."

Jane, in particular, talked about becoming comfortable with sharing her spiritual self with her patients. She made the following remarks:

> Spirituality is part of my practice, but it is a very personal part. Sharing your faith is not seen as a professional thing to do, and in nursing we are taught to be professional so I am hesitant to talk about it and admit to you that it is a part of my care. To me, it can be the true essence of everything — of life, of death. I do share my own beliefs if they are asking and they are feeling lost. I feel comfortable because I have my own beliefs together. People ask a lot of questions about the end, where they are going — especially if they haven't finished their business yet. But you do have to be careful. Sometimes, I just pray to myself.

## The emotional self

The nurses described what I have labeled emotional self-awareness. They talked about being "open to feeling the emotion of the moment, and being willing to share those feelings appropriately with others." During their careers, they had come to know themselves and to be sensitive to their emotions. Lana commented, "I always believed that if I couldn't recognize an emotion in myself like anger or sadness, how would I know it when I saw it in a patient?" Maureen concluded, "You have to know where you are at. If you don't know where you are coming from, how can you be available to help others?"

In summary, the importance of self-awareness — including awareness of the physical, spiritual, and emotional self — was identified and illustrated by the exceptionally competent nurses. This consciousness developed over time through experience and introspection. Identification of one's limitations and strengths were part of this process of self-discovery. A common sentiment is reflected in Jane's words. She said, "Working here, I have learned so much about cancer; but even more important, I have learned so much about myself. This no one can ever take away from me."

—

**ON DEVELOPING SELF-AWARENESS**

Mirror mirror in my friend,

tell me where this all will end?

What a marvelous mystery,

look at you, it's me I see!

—

### The significance of experiences with death

Many of the nurses' stories and my observations were about death, either the moment of death or the nurse's relationship with the dying patient and the patient's family. Although death is not a frequent topic of conversation and debate in society, these exceptionally competent nurses had thought about death and viewed helping a patient to a peaceful, dignified death as an important aspect of providing appropriate and successful nursing care. Though working with dying patients was described by the nurses as difficult, they did not seem to find this part of their job abhorrent; rather, they found it rewarding.

———

**THROUGH DEATH'S VALLEY TOWARD THE SUN**
The walk
down the hallway to the dying patient's room —
it seems so long.

The doors
to the dying patient's room —
so difficult to open.

But anyone
who has the strength
to take the walk,
who has the courage
to open those doors,

may discover an extraordinary opportunity
to learn about the things of life
that really matter.

———

The nurses I studied articulated and demonstrated comfort with the topic of death and dying, yet their experiences with this life process seemed to make a profound impact on them. Many of the nurses' most intense interactions with patients were with those who were seriously ill or dying. From encounters with the dying, the nurses learned lessons that changed the way they provided care to others. These challenging situations changed them both professionally and personally.

---

**BLENDING BORDERS**

There you are—
female, 32, a mother.

Here I stand—
female, 32, a mother.

By the nature of our similarities,
the borders of our realities blend.
When you hurt,
so do I,

When you cry,
so do I.

When you die,
so does a part of me.

---

## Moments of growth

Beyond their encounters with the dying, it appears that many of the significant practice moments reported by the exemplary nurses involved patients who shared similar circumstances with the nurse such as age, gender, or being parents to young children. The nurses wrote, at least in part, about how these experiences related to their own lives. Other memorable, critical nursing moments revolved around times when the nurses made a difference in someone else's life, when they learned something that changed their practice or their view of the world, and when they had an opportunity to share knowledge or insight with a colleague. During these significant practice moments when they taught others, the nurses also reported learning themselves. The exceptionally competent nurses were challenge seekers. It seems that many of these moments of growth came when they faced some of their greatest challenges.

## Touch, silence, and lightheartedness

The nursing actions of sharing the lighter side of life, participating in a dialogue of silence, and employing mutual touch are all means by which the exceptional nurses communicated with their patients. Sometimes nurses used these methods of communication while they were performing technical nursing interventions. On other occasions, these communications were the sole nursing activity of a nurse–patient encounter. By these means, the nurses let their patients know of their concern and respect for them. In a way, through these actions, the nurses communicated their beliefs and values to their patients.

A characteristic of these three communication modes is that they are all shared experiences, reciprocal in that both people are involved. Shared communication may be the means by which nurse–patient relationships are transformed into person-to-person relationships. Watson describes "human-to-human connectedness" and "transpersonal caring" and I believe that touch, silence, and lightheartedness may be ways by which these are achieved.[168]

According to Watson, in such circumstances "each person is touched by the human center of the other."[169] I suggest that when these moments occur there is an inter-human connection that leads to affirmation of value and transcendence of both the nurse and the patient. These moments are, as O'Banion and O'Connell describe, "Human encounters that have a diamond-like quality of brilliance and value and the potential to make one feel uplifted, completely understood, and transformed in some way."[170]

---

**PERSON TO PERSON**

In the beginning,
when I was a new nurse
standing in front of you
with trembling knees and
gleaming shoes and
textbook approaches,
I called you my patient.

Now,
I stand beside you,
I touch you,
I laugh with you,
I stay with you through silence,
and I call you by your name.

Our relationship is not simply
nurse to patient,
it is now
person to person.

---

*Motivation and satisfaction: A miracle circle*

The nurses' stories taught us something about how exemplary care-givers are motivated to continue to provide excellent care. Nursing is a positive and rewarding experience for these nurses. They expressed a high regard for their work. The intrinsic rewards they identified included feeling valued, and the opportunity for continued professional learning and personal growth, both of which they desired.

Many of the examples indicated that involvement in patient–nurse interactions within this context satisfied some of the nurses' priority needs. It seems that their actions initiated self-fulfilling reactions in cyclical fashion. As the exemplary nurses met the patients' needs in an exceptional way, they had their own needs fulfilled. Having been fulfilled themselves, the nurses were able — and perhaps even motivated — to continue to provide exceptional care to meet their patients' needs. In this way, nurses were both motivated by and found satisfaction in their work. The consequences became the basis for further exceptional care.

———

**THE MIRACLE CIRCLE CONTINUES**

My small gesture,
lovingly given,
causes you to feel valued.

When you feel important,
so do I.

Satisfied that I do make a difference,
I am motivated to continue to care for you
and for others.

———

## Confronting cancer: A shared experience

One of the incidental discoveries was a glimpse at the nature of cancer. The narratives provide an enhanced understanding of what it is like to confront this disease as a patient, a family member, and most clearly, as a nurse.

The stories reveal that cancer can involve intense human suffering and "chronic sorrow."[171] This disease shows no favoritism; it has the potential to affect anyone at any age or stage of life — no one, it seems, is immune.

Those affected by cancer and those around them are forced to confront their mortality. Part of the oncology experience seems to be grieving for oneself as well as for others. Confronting cancer causes people to lose their illusion of immortality, to recognize their vulnerability, and their lack of control over their health.

Providing care to those with many types of cancer is like fighting a war against death, disfigurement, and psychological and spiritual collapse — yours and the patient's. The nurses I studied showed us that, to be effective in this contest, nursing care must be complex, individualized, and delivered in a highly competent manner. The nurses fight for themselves and their own integrity as they fight for their patients. It is a shared experience.

From the stories, we can sense that the oncology milieu is one of intensity and urgency. At any moment, any one of the players could lose control, so there is a constant checking to see if they are all still within the threshold of normalcy.

Perhaps this ever-present sense of urgency, combined with the emotions that are part of each encounter to a greater or lesser extent, affected the nursing care the exemplary nurses gave. Such an environment reduces the "noise" in relationships and shortcuts are taken to establish meaningful inter-human connections quickly.

The oncology environment has the potential to be very stressful. Oncology nurses ride the waves of emotion with their patients. At any given moment, a nurse may be simultaneously experiencing the high of a disease in remission with one patient and the low of disease metastasized with another. It takes a very strong, self-aware person to be pulled and tugged in so many ways and to be able to withstand what would otherwise cause emotional and physical strain. Yet, if the nurses are able to stay with the struggle, as the exceptional ones do, they are forged like steel by the forces of emotions and the energy of experience. Rather than becoming brittle and immovable, exemplary nurses become stronger, preserved, and able to more easily withstand the forces in their environment.

---

**ON BEING A CANCER NURSE**
Every day you fight a battle against
physical, emotional, and spiritual collapse,
yours and your patients.

Each day is infused with an intensity,
a sense of urgency.
Waves of emotion wash over you
as you move from situation to situation.

At first you are never sure if
the next experience might be the big one,
the one that overwhelms you.
Eventually you find that from each
encounter you emerge stronger,
more sure of your abilities,
confident enough to carry on for the next day,
and probably the day after that.

---

## MESSAGES ADDRESSED TO EVERYONE

Some overarching insights emerged from the nurses' stories that may
have significance for people who work in other fields. These insights
are described below.

### Change: An opportunity for transcendence

Our lives are constantly changing. With each change come associated challenges that are opportunities for transcendence of self and others. For example, our level of wellness is not static and, with transitions in our states of well-being, new challenges are presented to self, family, and caregivers.

These challenges and changes in life, to self and others, are opportunities for transcendence. Perhaps the more serious the challenge or threat, the greater the possibilities for growth.

—

**ON THE CHANGES IN LIFE**

Change,
a part of your life and mine.

Embrace it.
Use it.
Grow through it.

—

## Touch: More than physical contact

Nurses and some other professionals, by the nature of the tasks prescribed by their roles, have implicit permission to physically touch their clients. Others are discouraged from physical contact with their clients for fear such gestures may be misinterpreted.

However, it seems that touch is more than physical contact between individuals. People can touch one another physically, but spiritual, emotional, and intellectual touch are also possibilities. People in each vocation may find one or more of these types of touch most appropriate to their work. For example, chaplains may communicate through spiritual alignment, psychologists through emotional contact, and teachers may touch their students intellectually through the sharing of information and cognitive challenges. People in human-services fields can let their clients know of their concern and respect for them by taking advantage of the communication opportunities provided by alternative approaches to touch.

---

**INTERPLAY OF THE MINDS**
When you share your
ideas and understandings with me,
it tells me that I
am important enough to
be trusted with something that is a part of you.

---

### The complexity of human interactions

Another broad understanding supported by this study is that human interaction is complex and sophisticated; different types of interaction — for example, verbal and non-verbal — usually occur simultaneously. People act as they react, and react as they act. The interpersonal process appears to be incessant, fluid, and non-linear.

Some of the most important elements in human interactions are the seemingly unheard and invisible. Although we do communicate through the well-recognized ways such as speech and gestures, we also communicate by laughing with others, touching them, and sharing silence with them.

If you touch others, remain present with them even in silence, or share with them in lightheartedness, you promote a sense of worth. In the larger view, this sense of self-worth in individuals may create a sense of worth in the community and, in turn, in society.

---

**HUMAN INTERACTIONS**
On closer inspection,
our interactions with others
are not as orderly
as I once thought.

---

## Transcendence: A shared process

Another important discovery concerns an increased understanding of transcendence. It appears to be a lifelong process. We are continually refined by our experiences, especially our interactions with others, with self, and perhaps with a higher entity. Being open to the promise that relationships offer may help us transcend to the highest level of human potential. We cannot transcend alone. To reach this premier state of being, we must be as open to receiving from others as we are open to giving to them.

—

**A JOURNEY SHARED**

We cannot transcend alone;
it is a shared journey.

As we transcend through our
experiences with others,
we open up the opportunity
for them to come along.

—

## An extended view of beauty

What is beauty? Time spent with the exceptional nurses helped me recognize that our dictionary and societal definitions of beauty are very limited. In the field, I saw beauty in many things that are not recognized generally as beautiful. As O'Banion and O'Connell say, "What is more beautiful than a man weeping, [or]...the eyes of someone welcoming death?"[172]

This extended view of beauty was important for the cancer nurses providing care. Once they redefined beauty, they saw the core of their patients — past what society labels as repulsive and unattractive. For similar reasons, others who work with people can benefit from an appreciation of beauty in more than its physical elements.

The following story written by Jane illustrates this redefinition of beauty.

I think the patient I will always remember is a woman named Heather. She was young, only 34, and she had flawless, olive skin and waist-length, thick, black hair. Heather was one of the most physically beautiful people I had ever cared for. Her recent diagnosis meant that her chemotherapy treatments had only just begun. I was the nurse responsible for administering her chemo. She was being treated with a combination of drugs known to cause hair loss.

Heather had just been hospitalized for her second course of chemotherapy. When I asked her how she had been since her last treatment, she talked about some nausea and mentioned that her hair was starting to fall out. She was noticing many strands on her pillow every morning. As the days went by, the hair loss became greater until it got so that she could pull her hair out by handfuls.

The night I remember, she rang her bell and asked if I could help remove the remainder of her hair. I did. We sat together on her bed with a green garbage bag between us stuffing it full of her beautiful hair. I was speechless. In fact, I couldn't believe what was happening. I felt so guilty having hair and being well.

When we were finished, we tied the bag closed. I looked right into her eyes, took both her hands and said, "Heather, I think you are still beautiful." I cried, and she comforted me. We hugged for awhile, and I took the bag and walked away.

—

**BEYOND BEAUTY**
You are a Goddess,
a beauty in body and spirit.
No matter how this disease ravishes you,
a beauty you will always be.


The temporary
and transient beauty
of your face,
your hair,
your body,
pale against the permanent beauty
of your soul.

—

## The power of storytelling

Stories are powerful ways to achieve insight into human interactions, partly because they are a natural means of communication. For me, they were important sources of understanding. An interview, no matter how unstructured, by its very nature imposes some limits on what is said and how it is expressed. Stories are liberating; they free the tellers so they can share what is important to them, and so they can analyze their experiences as they go along. Stories are rich with details about how the experience affected the storyteller. The following story written by Marie illustrates this well.

Linda was just 19 years old, and she had already lost her arm and shoulder to cancer. I was always amazed at how joyful and positive she was, and I thought, "This can't be for real." But it was. I learned Linda had lots of support at home. She was really close to her sister, and she had a strong religious conviction. I cared for her often over a period of about two years. Whenever we would have new patients with the same diagnosis as Linda, and she was around, she would offer to come and help me teach them about their disease. Using herself as a model, she would just whip off her shirt and show them her scars.

Toward the end, Linda met me in the hall and told me that her disease had spread and the doctors wanted her to try radiation treatments. I encouraged her to take the therapy; it was all I could do; she was only 19.

But for her, taking the radiation was wrong and she let me know that it was. I was stunned. I just kept shaking my head and saying in disbelief, "You are not going to try?" I felt upset because she wasn't fighting it. The nurse in me wanted to do something for her. I didn't want to lose her. It would have been easier for me to be more palliative with her if she had been in my age group, but she was only a teenager.

When she saw I was falling apart, Linda took me aside, put her arm around me and said, "No, Marie — it has just spread too much. I can't do this any longer. I'm okay. I know I'm going to die, and I am okay. with that." I was shattered.

A few weeks later, we had a call from the nurses in Linda's community. It's a couple of hours drive from here. They wanted to learn how to look after her at home so she could be with her family until the end. I asked to be the one to go to the community and teach the nurses what they needed to know. Though I was eight months pregnant with my first child, I wanted to be the one to do something for her.

About 15 minutes into the teaching session with the nurses, Linda showed up. She wasn't well. She was thin and pale, but she looked at me and said, "Here I am, Marie. I wanted to come today and be your model like I've always been."

Then the class was over, and she had to go. I wasn't coping very well with the goodbye because I knew it would be our last. Again she nurtured me. I will never forget what she said…She said, "Marie, it's okay — in fact, it's kind of exciting. Here you are going off on a new journey of motherhood, and I'm off on a journey of my own. We are both going to be just fine."

I was so preoccupied driving home. It was true. I was off to become a mom and she was off to…I didn't know for sure to where, or to what — but she did.

As well, telling stories may have a cathartic effect, and it can be a further method of increasing self-awareness of the teller. It appears that storytelling helps the teller as well as the listener understand an experience. This is clearly illustrated in Julie's comments:

I just want to say thanks for helping me open up a part of me I could have shared in no other way but by writing my stories. There was something so liberating about sitting down with a blank page.

## WHAT I LEARNED ABOUT EXEMPLARY NURSING

Exceptional nursing practice is more than being technically competent. It is being self-aware and communicating with patients person-to-person through touch, silence, and sharing the lighter side of life. These actions involve nurses sharing part of themselves with the patients, and encouraging the patients to share themselves with the nurses.

Exemplary nurses have well-developed nursing philosophies that become their blueprints for action. Important elements of these philosophies include a reverence for life and respect for the value of each individual. These nurses have become self-aware and have developed their philosophies at least partly through interaction with patients with whom they have identified closely, through teaching others, and through experiences with death.

Exemplary nurses seem to be both motivated by their work and draw satisfaction from it, especially by the opportunity to feel valued for what they do and by the chance for personal and professional growth. Exceptional nursing practice includes sharing the disease experience with the patients, struggling and growing with them, and using unfortunate circumstances as an opportunity for both the nurse and patient to achieve transcendence.

Exemplary nursing care is good for the nurse and the patient, and it can often still be achieved within the constraints of the complex and dynamic health-care milieu. The foundation for exemplary nursing care seems to be in the nurses' willingness to establish connections with their patients. These connections can be achieved in part through certain attitudes and small acts on the part of the nurse. Further, a nurse-patient connection can occur in brief encounters in the emergency room or in longer-term relationships on a palliative care unit. Askinazi notes that "this connection is a gift for the patient as much as of the caregiver…. There is the potential in certain patient-caregiver relationships of something transcendental."[173]

Nurses who are truly exemplary embrace the experience of inter-dependence, willingly entwining themselves with others, learning and sharing with colleagues, patients, family members, and students. The secret of the satisfying caregiver-other relationships is the trans-forming potential of caring. Satisfied nurses who connect with, and journey with, others in caring relationships are, potentially, positively affected by the experience. They may, if they allow it, learn many life lessons and find themselves changed by caring. Let me illustrate with a story from a nurse I met at a conference.

A year or so ago, I was working nights. My patient became increasingly restless and agitated. He had a progressive dementia, and he was more disturbed than any patient I had cared for in my 25 years or more of nursing. That night, he required two-to-one nursing care.

Around 0300 hours, the other nurse I was working with observed that, in spite of his verbal lashing out, he had never once cursed. She remarked that he must not have "bad" words in his normal vocabulary because usually what is in a mind comes out in confusion. The night wore on with our patient experiencing agitation, yelling, and extreme restlessness. He would bite his own hands and arms and grab on to anything near him. We began to wonder if we could ever help him rest. I remember feeling helpless and hopeless.

Then I heard him repeat a series of words in a garbled fashion and recognized the words of an old hymn. I began to sing the hymn, and immediately he became quiet. The change was instantaneous and profound. The other nurse was able to leave for a break while I sat beside him singing every hymn I could remember.

As long as the hymns were sung, the patient rested. (She added a side note saying that it was a good thing she was a PK — a preacher's kid — and because of this, she knew a lot of hymns). We later found out that the man had been a lay pastor, and perhaps this explained his reaction to my music.

I loved being his nurse because none of the usual textbook interventions worked. He required flexible, creative nurses who were not afraid to try the unconventional and who were willing to keep trying until we could find a way to connect with him and his needs. Large doses of artificial sedation made no difference. Somewhere in the deepest levels of this man's mind, our presence through music and just being near touched him. It was a profound night because all my years of training and education came down to the simple singing of a song.

—

**CHANGED**

Caring for you
has left an unforgettable impression
on my soul.

—

Askinazi writes: "There's a mystery to nursing, a secret energy that forms in the nurse-patient relationship. It is the experience of caring, and the memories of these experiences, which lead to confidence, self-esteem and energy."[174] In writing about their own experiences with the "mystery of the nurse-patient relationship," Hagerty and Patusky conclude: "[We] have glimpsed instead a much wilder, more gripping kind of feeling that is both exhilarating and dynamic. The secret of the caregiver-patient relationship is the transforming potential of caring."[175]

Nurses predictably and regularly interact meaningfully with people facing some the most demanding and emotional moments of their lives — bringing forth life, fighting disease, accepting death, or tolerating disintegration of body or spirit. For anyone who desires to engage in meaningful human relationships, nursing provides the perfect avenue. Through these "intimate human connections, nurses are able to share their gifts with the community and the world."[176] As nurses give of themselves, they are affirmed and come to know that they have value. Career satisfaction is the potential result — nurses who can sincerely say, "I love my work!"

The exemplary care-career satisfaction cycle is also important for the patient because of the potential positive influence on quality of care. Nurses who describe themselves as sure they had made the right career choice are also more likely to provide nursing care that was considered by their colleagues to be of exemplary quality. In other words, when nurses do their work well, they are more likely to be professionally fulfilled and to continue the positive cycle of excellent caregiving.[177] Such nurses have discovered that nursing is more.

I believe there is power and promise embedded in exemplary nursing care. The stories and poems presented in this book expose the often hidden, yet invaluable, contribution made by clinical nurses. The nurses' words illustrate the challenge of living with cancer and of caring for people with this disease.

For the profession of nursing, this work has contributed to the growing body of knowledge that the profession can consider its own. Some of the essential features of exceptional nursing practice have been explored and described.

There are many more insights that could be drawn from these stories and field notes. Probably the most important discoveries will be made by practicing clinicians — nurses who read this book and examine the ideas within the context of their own practice.

What a difference each one of you makes. As you magnify this magic by your numbers, together you become a brilliant light in the world. Each one of you is a small light; each individual makes the world for the others a little better — and when you join with other like-minded people together, your light is strong and you make the world a better place for everyone. You make the world brighter and more love filled and, in doing so, you SHINE. I honour you and thank you. Well done my colleagues — well done.

---

### NURSING IS MORE
Nursing is much more
than procedures
and policies.

It is getting inside
someone's mind,
and knowing what will make them whole.

It is taking a risk
and helping someone
do something they need to do, but can't.

It is campaigning
for something you know someone needs
even when they are unaware.

It is jeopardizing
the certain
to attain the essential.

---

—

**LESSONS LEARNED ON BECOMING AND BEING EXEMPLARY**

Touch others,
physically, emotionally, intellectually, and spiritually.
Learn to use silence,
it provides a powerful means of communication.

Approach life lightheartedly,
lightness can be shared even in the darkest seasons.

Focus on the potential,
yours and others.

Embrace change,
it is an opportunity for transcendence.
Find work that you enjoy,
that makes you feel valued and challenged.

Study people carefully,
in doing so you will learn much about yourself.

Determine what you know,
and seek chances to teach it to others.

Discover what you believe,
and live it with confidence.

Appreciate others,
and pursue opportunities to contribute to their happiness.

Realize that you are not perfect,
and accept that you probably will never be.

Know your strengths,
and blend these with the strengths of those you meet.

See beauty,
for it is all around in forms not instantly recognizable.

Be as open to receiving as you are to giving,
this is a gift to others as well as to yourself.

Seek challenges,
and enjoy the privilege of learning from them.

Tell your stories,
for they are you.

Share your journey,
you cannot sparkle alone.

—

# *appendix*

## RESEARCH DESIGN
## AND METHODOLOGY

This appendix describes the research design and methodology used in the study that formed the basis for this book. Beginning with a brief exploration of the nature of qualitative inquiry, a case is made for its use in nursing 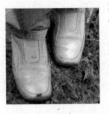 investigations that focus on human experience. The methodology used in the study, hermeneutic phenomenology, is discussed. Specifics about the study participants, approaches to data collection, and methods of data analysis are described. Techniques used to maintain data trustworthiness, assumptions made, delimitations and limitations of the study, and ethical considerations are included.

### QUALITATIVE INQUIRY

This qualitative study was designed to explore aspects of exemplary nursing care. The goal of this type of study is the accurate portrayal and interpretation of what is being investigated from the participants' viewpoints.[178] Benner and Wrubel maintain that this approach is appropriate when studying human experience in complex, elusive, and still largely unexplored areas such as exemplary nursing care.[179]

The assumptions, premises, and expectations of qualitative research are most congruent with the traditional values of nursing as a personalized, intimate, and holistic human service. Qualitative research attempts to grasp the essential features of phenomena so the essence of the person, object, or experience is revealed.[180]

To accomplish this goal, qualitative researchers enter the participant's world to gather information first-hand through oral and written accounts, symbols, language, and observations. As Loiselle and Profetto-McGrath define this approach, it is characterized by a research design that is flexible and emergent; the researcher may reformulate and expand the study and approaches used as the study proceeds.[181] These design decisions reflect what the researcher has learned as the study takes place.

The goal of this study was an exploration of the nature of exemplary nursing. To succeed in such a quest, a method that encourages close contact with participants in their worlds is necessary in order to see the context in which they work and to view exemplary care in a holistic manner.

### HERMENEUTIC PHENOMENOLOGY

The terms methodology and methods are often confused. Methodology refers to the philosophic framework, general orientation to life, the view of knowledge, and fundamental assumptions associated with a certain research approach. Method is the steps or procedures for gathering and analyzing research data.[182] In some ways, methodology is the theory behind the method. Van Manen adds that the methods that are used need to be developed in response to the research question and must be congruent with the methodology chosen.[183] The first step is the determination of the methodology. Once the methodology is clear, the research methods to be used become evident. The methodology for this study was hermeneutic phenomenology.

Hermeneutics is an approach to studying humans that is rooted in the philosophy, and based on the views, of phenomenologist Martin

216

Heidegger.[184] According to van Manen, hermeneutics is the interpretive study of the expressions of lived experiences in the attempt to determine the meaning embodied in them.[185]

Phenomenology is the study and description of human phenomena. As Laverty explains, the terms phenomenology and hermeneutics are often used interchangeably; however, phenomenology focuses on the "lived experience" whereas hermeneutics refers to the interpretation of the experience.[186] Gaut used the two words in combination, defining hermeneutic phenomenology as the interpretation of concealed meaning within a phenomenon.[187] It becomes difficult, and perhaps unnecessary, to differentiate between hermeneutic (the interpretation) and phenomenology (the description) since, at one level, a description is itself an interpretation.

A basic tenet of phenomenology is that each person is unique and possesses potential. Researchers who pursue phenomenological studies ask the question: "What is the essence of this phenomenon as experienced by these people?" Phenomenologists assume that this essence can be described and understood.

Merleau-Ponty explains that the word essence should not be mystified. He notes that essence may be understood as a description of a phenomenon. The essence is "a linguistic description that is holistic and analytical, evocative and precise, unique and universal, powerful and sensitive."[188] According to van Manen, "The essence or nature of the experience has been adequately described in language if the description reawakens or shows us the lived quality and significance of the experience in a fuller or deeper manner."[189]

Van Manen describes the characteristics of phenomenological research. It begins in the world of those being studied. Lived experience is the starting point and end point of phenomenological research. "The aim of phenomenology is to transform lived experience into a textual expression of its essence."[190] In van Manen's view, the phenomenological investigation does not result in a theory with which the world can be explained; rather, it offers plausible insights that bring us all in more direct contact with the world.[191]

The focus of phenomenology is on meaning, and the goal is to explicate meanings as we experience them in our everyday existence. Hermeneutic phenomenology is a human science which studies persons. It is not interested in the generalizable; it is a philosophy of the unique, interested in what is essentially not replicable.[192]

Heidegger describes phenomenological research as a minding, a heading, a caring attunement.[193] To van Manen, it is "the attentive practice of thoughtfulness."[194] The latter cautions, "To do hermeneutic phenomenology is to attempt to accomplish the impossible: to construct a full interpretive description of some aspect of the life world, and yet to remain aware that lived life is always more complex than an explication of meaning can reveal."[195] Despite this cautionary note, an attempt at the impossible still has merit. Though a description can never be complete, it does bring us closer to an understanding of a phenomenon.

There is no step-by-step method for doing phenomenological research. Merleau-Ponty advises that the only way to learn it, and understand it, is to do it.[196] Gadamer, supporting this position, writes that the method of hermeneutic phenomenology is that there is no method.[197]

Although there is no specific method, there is a tradition, a set of guides and recommendations. Phenomenologists search for "the critical moments of inquiry." As van Manen states, "such moments depend on the interpretive sensitivity, inventiveness, thoughtfulness, scholarly tact, and writing talent of the human science researcher."[198] Benner and Wrubel maintain that the products of hermeneutic phenomenology inquiry may include thick description, paradigm cases, exemplars, and thematic analysis — all of which explicate meaning and ways of being.[199]

The hermeneutic phenomenology approach in this investigation contributes to our understanding of the experience and it can inform the way we think and feel about exemplary nursing care. In brief, what this chosen methodology contributes is the rich contextualized detail of this human experience. Table 1 summarizes the elements of hermeneutic phenomenology.

TABLE 1: **ELEMENTS OF HERMENEUTIC PHENOMENOLOGY**

Derived from the philosophy of phenomenology

Behavior studied in context, direct contact with participants

Based on actual realities of people as they live through their experiences

Emphasizes meaning, lived experience, textual expression of the essence

Meaning guides behavior

Goal — discover meaning and further understanding of phenomena

Does not attempt to generalize

Analysis and data collection occur simultaneously

Interviews are main method of data collection

Interpretation of data aims to unveil hidden meaning

Analysis generates exemplars, cases, and themes

Data are left intact; researchers search for the essence

Literature review serves as background meaning for analysis

Validity is checked by participants responding to textual expression of the essence

Provides rich detail that can inform practice

Study dependent on creative insights of the researcher

## RESEARCH METHOD

This section describes the research project that informed this book: the participants, methods of data collection and analysis, trustworthiness, assumptions, delimitations and limitations, and ethical considerations.

## Participants

The general principles employed when selecting a group of participants in qualitative research are appropriateness and adequacy.[200] Appropriateness refers to the degree to which the choice of informants and method of selection fits the purpose of the study. Adequacy is related to sufficiency and quality of data. If the sample is "efficient," (that is, the respondents freely provide insightful and numerous comments and examples, and there are many opportunities of meaningful observations), the size of the sample can be small and still be adequate.[201] It is desirable to have informants who are articulate, reflective, patient with the process, and willing to share their views with the researcher. To ensure appropriateness and adequacy, the researcher must have control over the sample.

My goal was to locate a group of nurses who were considered by their peers to be exceptionally competent practitioners. I had narrowed my clinical study area to oncology, so I attempted to find oncology nurses who met my criterion.

After gaining access to a nursing unit in a large, urban care facility where the majority of the patients had cancer, I distributed letters through the hospital mail system to all registered nurses (RNs) who worked on that unit. In the letter, I introduced myself and my research and asked them to independently construct a list of names of nurses who worked on their unit who they believed were exceptionally competent. This method of selecting exceptional practitioners had been used in studies of expert nurses,[202] and excellent physicians.[203] Benner and Wrubel report that expert nurses are easily identified by asking for nominations from their colleagues.[204]

To clarify for the nominating nurses what I meant by "exceptionally competent," I asked them to consider those nurses who they would choose to have care for them or their family members if they had cancer. In my view, this was the essential criterion, the one that would encompass many of the important aspects of excellent nursing practice. As a side note, as I have explained my research method to groups of nurses across Canada in more recent years, this method of selecting exemplary nurses has received the approval of many audiences. When I say, "I am sure right now each of you could think of those nurses you work with that you would want to care for you" there is always a chorus of the affirmative responses from the audience. This gives me confidence in this participant selection process.

For the study, the nurses were free to nominate themselves and any other nurses from their unit that they believed met the criterion. To increase their level of comfort in participating in this exercise, the nurses were assured that no nurse would ever know for certain if he or she had been nominated, except for the nurses who were eventually invited to participant in the study. This was facilitated by choosing the actual study participants randomly from the list of nominated nurses.

The written, anonymous, nominations were placed by each nurse into a sealed envelope which was collected by the unit manager and delivered unopened to me. I did not know from whom each list of nominees had come. During the three-week period between the distribution of the letter requesting nominations and the submission of the nomination lists, I was available on the nursing unit at specified times to answers questions and concerns regarding the nomination process. There were very few questions, but this face time on the nursing unit did help the staff to get to know me and increased the comfort level between us which proved to be very helpful during the data collection phase.

After the nomination phase ended, I compiled the names. Of the 30 nurses who were asked for nominations, 25 responded with a list of nominees. There was remarkable consistency among the names of nominees. The same names appeared on most of the nomination forms to such an extent that I felt comfortable that I had a pool of exceptionally competent nurses from which to choose study partici-pants. The eventual master list contained the names of nurses who were nominated at least 20 times. From this list, six nurses were randomly chosen to participate in the study.

The nurses who were selected as potential participants were sent letters formally inviting them to be part of the study. Those interested in becoming study participants signed an informed consent from and returned it to me. All the nurses who were approached agreed to be in the study. The names of other nurses who were nominated at least 20 times but who were not randomly selected from the master list were kept in reserve. By the end of the study, two more nurses were added to the sample for a total of eight participants.

Who were the exceptional nurses who were studied? A composite picture of the nurse participants emerges in the following description of the daily routine on the nursing unit where the study was based. The nurses featured in this scenario are the eight study participants. This illustration serves several purposes. First, it includes a depiction of the nurses studied, letting you see the pertinent demographics of the study participants. Though they were all unique, it is interesting that their demographics overlapped in many spheres. Second, this description provides an example of the routine followed by a clini-cal oncology nurse working on the study unit. This affords you an understanding of the context and setting in which oncology nurses work. While no two days, or two shifts, or two nurses were exactly the same, there were similarities that make it possible for this com-posite description of an average day to be constructed. To help the reader get to know the participants, their average day is described in the following section.

## An average day on the unit

It's 0700 hours and the eight RNs participating in the study (Jane, Maureen, Marie, Julie, Lana, Peter, Moria, and Cindy) were gathered around a table in the conference room to listen to a tape-recorded report on the condition of each patient staying on their unit. The report is provided by the nurses who are just finishing the night shift. As I look about the room, I am surprised at how alert the staff members look. I wonder how they can exude so much energy at this hour of the morning.

They have dressed thoughtfully. One is wearing a peach-colored uniform with a lacy collar that she crocheted herself. Another wears a bright smock over her scrubs. "We need a little color around here," she chirps when one of her colleagues comments on her uniform. As they wait for the nurse in charge to enter the conference room and begin report, the nurses enthusiastically exchange tales about their personal lives.

They are all women, except one, and the oldest of them has not quite reached her sixth decade — the youngest is 29. All but one are married. Most of the married nurses have children varying in age from toddler to young adult. Each nurse has worked on the study unit for a minimum of two years; the most senior has 11 years of oncology experience. For one woman, nursing is her third career. She had been a teacher and school principal before becoming an oncology nurse two years ago. One nurse had 20 years experience in the operating room before transferring to the cancer unit two years before. Stories of juggling the needs of their children, spouses, community, and other commitments permeate the pre-report conversations.

The charge nurse enters, and the air becomes quiet and professional. Outside the closed door of the conference room, the night-shift nurses hurry to finish their tasks — such as making notes on each patient's chart and answering call bells. Report begins. The day nurses and I listen to the jargon-laden details of each patient's condition.

"Mr. Jakes in room 10 slept well and needs to have a urine specimen collected this morning. Mrs. Kennedy in room 12 is due at the x-ray department today, and her intravenous bag only has 100 mL to be absorbed. Mr. Millright in room 14 experienced a lot of pain during the night and needed analgesic medication every three hours. He is due for a scan today. His daughter called and she was very tearful."

The report goes on until details of each patient have been recounted. The nurses have carefully recorded the pertinent information regarding the patients assigned to them and, as the voice on the tape machine says, "Have a great day shift," the nurses gather their notes, place them in uniform pockets, and set off to do morning rounds. As they leave the conference room, the nurse in charge calls out words of encouragement saying, "We are short one nurse today. Marg called in sick and they can't replace her. It looks like we have a lot of heavy patients. Let's work together!"

Each nurse is assigned to give care to a group of patients. The patients who are critically ill or close to death stay in private rooms; others may be in semi-private accommodations. The number of patients in a nurse's assignment varies depending on the amount of care each patient requires. Jane has six patients today, while Maureen has only one very ill man to care for.

Morning rounds consist of a quick check on the patients to meet any immediate needs such as toileting assistance, replacement of intravenous bags that are low, or realignment of people who are uncomfortable. During rounds, priorities are set and plans are made by each nurse for the care to be given that day. The common morning rounds questions addressed to patients include, " What time would you like your bath? Are you expecting any visitors today? What is your pain level — should we try your pain pills every three hours? How is your breathing?"

The morning proceeds smoothly — a series of breakfast, baths, and personal hygiene interventions punctuated with administration of medications and ongoing assessment of each patient's physical and emotional status. Interruptions by doctors seeking information, family members needing reassurance, and colleagues requiring assistance are all incorporated readily into the routine. "Routine," Peter explains, "is part of each day. You need it to make sure certain tasks get done.... It gives structure — backbone to the more creative parts of nursing."

I am fascinated by the perpetual motion. It seems the nurses never stop moving, talking, questioning, listening, lifting, and writing. Often they do two or more tasks simultaneously. Finally, they take a break. We gather at the elevator to go to the cafeteria for lunch. The nurses take their meal breaks in two shifts. Before leaving the unit, each nurse reports to another nurse who is staying behind, making certain all patients will be cared for in their absence.

At lunch, I find out more about these nurses. They have such busy lives outside their work. For example, one collects dolls, one sews, one golfs and swims, one paints, one enjoys the outdoors and nature, one plays four musical instruments, one teaches Sunday school and is president of her community league, and one has three preschoolers. Animated discussions tell me they are as passionate about their hobbies and interests as they are about nursing. In conversation, Lana says, "I believe that we can be better nurses if we have something else in our lives besides nursing." Everyone agrees with her.

We talk about their education. "Where did you study nursing?" I ask. They have all completed a registered nurse diploma program. Two have finished post-basic bachelor's degrees in nursing in addition to their diplomas. Lifelong learning is a value each nurse expresses, and they talk about the importance of "staying current" by attending conferences, reading professional journals, and asking questions.

Our break is short because there are medications that are due to be administered, Mrs. Jones needs to be repositioned, and the physiotherapist is coming to show them how to use a new patient-lifting device that will "save their backs." As we proceed toward the elevator to return to the nursing unit, they make the transition in their speech and demeanor back to the world of work.

The afternoon goes by quickly. It seems most of the plans made this morning have been modified, and the nurses are now being driven primarily by the request of patients and physicians. There is a flurry of activity just before shift change at 1500 hours as the day nurses try to squeeze in time to complete the charted notes on each patient and to tape-record report for the nurses who will be working the afternoon shift. Simultaneously, they greet visitors, explain changes in each patient's status to doctors and family members, and answer patient call bells with grace and cheerfulness. I could best describe the afternoon as "endless interruptions," yet they all maintain their poise.

There is a detectable sense of relief in the air as the afternoon shift nurses begin to arrive. The day nurses are starting to look fatigued. Their once-fresh uniforms are wrinkled and stained, and their steps are a little slower. As they put on their coats to go home, they talk about how tired they are, but they still smile. There is a sense of achievement; the team has pulled together, and they collectively feel satisfied with the quality of care they were able to give. Getting on the elevator to leave, Julie turns back. She has forgotten to tell her replacement nurse that Mr. Yin asked for ice cream for supper, and she wants to make sure he gets it — she promised.

## Data collection

To be true to the tenets of hermeneutic phenomenology, I chose data-gathering approaches that ventured into the participants' worlds, thereby studying human experience in context. I sought to find ways of reaching into the realities of the exceptional nurses to try to capture how they were experiencing and functioning in their work worlds. By choosing to use a combination of field-based methods including observation, in-depth interviews (conversations), and narrative exchange, I endeavored to get a comprehensive view of exceptional nursing practice.

Each nurse was studied individually. Observations were conducted with each participant over a period of approximately 40 hours, covering a variety of shifts and days of the week. Following or during the observation period, I held an in-depth interview that was more like a conversation with each participant.

After a period of retreat from the study site and initial analysis of the data, further conversations were conducted with some of the participants. In addition, the process of narrative exchange was initiated with all participants. This resulted in several supplemental contacts with most participants.

### Observation

From the beginning of my field work, I recorded my observations, thoughts, and insights in a research journal. Throughout this discussion of data collection methods, I include excerpts from this log as I think they most clearly communicate the details of the process undertaken.

My field notes were not as precise in their execution as I first imagined they would be. I did make discoveries and change my data collection tactics as I proceeded. However, I always tried to remain very aware of what was happening, or where my research was leading me. I believe the result of my openness to letting go and learning from others is an accurate and intimate portrayal of exceptional nursing practice.

One example of a change in my approach was a move from a participant-observer role to that of an observer-participant. The following journal entry details this transition.

It's 0600 hours and I struggle out of bed and put on my uniform to start another day of observations on the unit. As I drive toward the hospital and think about my plans for the day, I am glad I made the decision to observe rather than participate.

When I started the study, I imagined being like a second set of hands to the nurse I was observing — a participant-as-observer in textbook terms. But it just wasn't working. Sure, I was a "big help" since I am an oncology nurse too, but I was missing the action as I ran here and there delivering cups of tea or answering call bells. The nurses were confused about what I could and couldn't do (as I wasn't an employee, I was limited to volunteer roles); in fact, even I got confused sometimes. It's hard to remember I'm a researcher and not a nurse right now.

Being an observer-participant is better for my purposes. Now I'm just like a shadow; I stay quiet and out of the way, and I am surprised that no one even seems to notice me anymore. I think what I am observing is more real somehow; the nurses aren't performing for me anymore. They seem to have forgotten that I am even there.

Pearsall was one of the first to describe the role continuum for participant-observers, a continuum ranging from complete observer to complete participant.[205] According to Pearsall, in the observer-as-participant role, the researcher remains "detached and objective" and observation takes precedence. Alternatively, in the participant-as-observer role, close interpersonal relationships may develop with informants as the observer enters the social and cultural milieu of the participants.[206] The observer-participant role was most appropriate during the observation phase of the study; however, during the interviews and narrative exchanges, I became more interactive and intimate with the participants.

My observations were primarily of nurse-patient encounters. However, as this entry from my research journal describes, I did expand the scope of my observations as the study progressed.

I find I am observing the nurses everywhere we go — not just with patient interactions, but also when they are on breaks, in conferences, or attending rounds. Perhaps because they know I'm a nurse, they seem really comfortable with me and invite me to follow them into the medication room and some of their other "insider" spaces.

When appropriate, brief notes regarding the observations were made during the shift. Notes were recorded away from the scene of the interactions. At the completion of every observation shift, I elaborated upon these comments in my research journal.

I originally planned to keep a separate diary to log research-related ideas, fears, mistakes, confusions, breakthroughs, and problems. However, it became difficult to separate feelings and observations, so both process items and the details of the research observations were documented in the same journal.

I believe that my experience as an oncology nurse prepared me to make meaningful observations and also to know how to observe without compromising patient care or making anyone uncomfortable. This journal entry summarizes that struggle.

I worried a lot at first about whether or not I would be sensitive enough to what was happening to know when it was in the patient's or nurse's best interest to step out and not observe a particular moment. I didn't want to prevent something important from being said, or make anyone feel uncomfortable. Today, I just stayed outside the room when Mr. Kim had his enema. Somehow I felt he would be uncomfortable with me there, too. Afterwards the nurse thanked me for being so tactful. When the mother of that girl with the brain tumour started to cry with the nurse I was observing, I just backed away to give them the private moment they needed.

The observation phase of the study provided very rich data. I wrote in my journal,

> I am so glad that I decided to include observations in data collection. The nurses can't always put into words what they were doing and why. They couldn't tell me, but their actions showed me. The looks, tears, hugs, smiles, hesitations, or playful touches couldn't have been captured except by the camera of my mind. A lot of exceptional nursing care is in the non-verbal.

Levine advises that some things can only be learned by wading in slowly, from the direct experience of the ocean lapping against our bodies.[207] The observational phase of this study allowed me this opportunity to wade in and experience the oncology world the way the nurses were experiencing it.

## Interviews

The interviews — or, more appropriately, the conversations — conducted as part of data collection were open dialogues about the meaning of exceptional practice and each nurse's experiences in oncology nursing. To encourage the informal nature of these encounters, they were held in places that the participants identified as most convenient and comfortable for them. Most of the conversations were taped with the permission of the nurses, and the tapes were transcribed. The conversations used an unstructured approach with open-ended questions. This seemed to unlock the idea gate and encouraged the participants to tell their stories in their own words. Polit and Hungler counsel that, "Imposing structure on the research situation by deciding in advance exactly what questions to ask restricts the portion of the subject's experience that will be revealed."[208]

I found the unstructured method resulted in long discussions filled with accounts of exceptional moments from the work lives of the nurses. Through their stories, they freely shared their beliefs about oncology nursing, their feelings about what they do and why it is effective, and their attitudes about their work. Most conversations lasted between one and two hours.

### Narrative exchange

According to Benner, experienced nurses can readily bring to mind clinical situations that altered their approach to patient care. She called these paradigm cases.[209] A systematic study of these cases can reveal embedded knowledge. Following the observation and conversation phases, I turned to collecting the nurses' written stories of their most memorable practice moments — their paradigm cases.

During the data collection phase, I had written in my journal my own transformational patient-care experiences. As I asked study participants to record their stories for me, I became interested in the idea of narrative exchange, a written dialogue between the researcher and the participants. In my research journal, I wrote of this idea.

> Today I had an interesting idea. What about talking to the nurses through my own stories? Sometimes hearing someone else's experience really triggers your own memory, and if someone is open with you, it encourages openness in return. Maybe if I share my stories with them, they will be willing to reciprocate. If we are really in this together like I have said we are, exposing part of me may liberate part of them. This is more like doing research with them instead of on them or to them. I think I will call this process narrative exchange.

The narrative exchange data-collection process involved me offering each participant a letter and several of my own narratives, suggesting that they too might have stories of exceptional practice moments they would be willing to share. In the letter, I asked, "Who are the patients you still remember? Can you recall particular moments with them that were most important or perhaps changed you or your practice?"

The response was varied. One nurse wrote about a single critical moment, while others wrote many pages about detailed exchanges with their past patients. They all offered striking examples of exceptional nursing practice. The knowledge revealed through the stories was contextualized and personal. Each story was unique — rich with its own cadence, style, personality, and wisdom.

As Ellis and Flaherty believe, research methods need to "shrink the distance" between the research participants and their experience.[210] The writing of stories offers this opportunity. Ellis and Flaherty go on to say that, "writing stories is a conversation with self and through this conversation we come to know ourselves."[211] Narrative exchange is a method that can make a lived experience understandable to self and others and a means by which this understanding can be communicated.

As the nurses wrote their stories, many stated in notes or conversations with me how meaningful the writing experience was for them. In a card, Marie wrote,

> I would like to thank you for asking me to share some of my memories. After reading your memories, I wanted to begin to write immediately, but I couldn't. My special moments were hard to retrieve. Many of them were difficult, some were sad, but all left a deep imprint on my perception and on the way I do things today. This was indeed a valuable exercise for me; like you, I relived some successes and some fears too, all of which have produced the nurse I am now. I feel truly blessed by what I have taken from these experiences, for what I've become because of them, and for what I have been able to do for others.

Julie addressed these comments to me,

> I just wanted to say thanks for helping me open up a
> part of me that I could have shared in no other way but
> by writing my stories. There was something so liberat-
> ing about sitting down with a blank page. I just sat and
> talked to the paper, and to you. The memories just came
> flooding back. Perhaps I've guarded them, protected
> them like keepsakes stored away in a secret chest. Now
> I'm so happy to have the chance to share them. It has
> helped me see the whole picture of my practice.

The use of observations, conversation-like interviews, and narrative
exchange as described was in keeping with the data-collection methods
appropriate to hermeneutic phenomenology. These data-collection
methods produced abundant data to be analyzed and understood.

## Data analysis

In qualitative research, most times data collection and analysis occur
simultaneously in a spiral of increasing complexity rather than alone
in a linear continuum. As the researcher ascends through the various
levels in the spiral, new dimensions of understanding are uncovered
and new questions emerge that expand and support the findings.

Polit and Hungler note that, "There is no systematic, universally
accepted rules for analyzing and presenting qualitative data."[212] However, in approaching data analysis, there were certain principles that
I sought to uphold. For example, I wanted to be true to the nurses
who participated. To me, this meant including the context and, as
much as possible, using the nurses' words — giving them a chance
to express themselves in their own voices. Consequently, I used the
nurses' stories and comments verbatim throughout the reporting of
findings. Care was taken not to fragment the experiences because to
do so would "distort that which they seek to describe."[213] The intact

stories facilitate knowledge being revealed to the reader without forcing interpretation.

There is no step-by-step method for analyzing phenomenological research data. As van Manen states, "The critical moments of inquiry are ultimately elusive to systematic explication. Indentifying and communicating such moments may depend on the interpretive sensitivity, inventiveness, thoughtfulness, scholarly tact, and writing talent of the human-science researcher."[214] The aim of phenomenological analysis is to "construct an animated, evocative description (text) of human actions, behaviors, intentions, and experiences as we meet them in their life world."[215] It focuses on describing essential themes; it is "a thoughtful, reflective grasping of the special significance of this or that particular experience...bringing into nearness that which tends to be obscure."[216] Anderson summarizes, claiming the intent of phenomenology is "not to build grand theories of nursing but to understand the lived experience of people."[217]

However, to discover the meaning of human experiences, some analysis is necessary. Guidance as to how this discovery can be accomplished is provide by Oiler.[218] Oiler suggests that analysis begins when the researcher reads all descriptions to obtain "a feel for them."[219] During this reading, researchers attempt to hold in abeyance their presuppositions about the phenomena so that the phenomena can be seen as they are, not as they are reflected through preconceptions.

Next, from each source, significant statements and phrases are identified, and meanings are formulated from these. The meanings are organized into themes which are displayed as a description of the experience. Uncovered themes provide the essence of the experience. To achieve validation, the researcher returns the descriptions to the participants for feedback.[220]

### Multi-dimensional analysis

I followed the Oiler process and eventually designed a multi-dimensional analysis of the data. One part of the analysis does not necessarily follow another in a step-wise manner, rather each is important and somewhat independent of the others. While each analysis makes an important contribution to the overall understanding of exceptionally competent nursing practice, one can appreciate an individual analysis for its own unique characteristics.

The first analysis was provided by the participants themselves as they shared their memories and comments with me. They offered personal reflections and meaningful insights on their descriptions of events. As the nurses wrote their stories and talked to me, they would often say, "What I learned from this was...," or "I think I did this to...." As the study progressed, the nurses reflected on their own descriptions and actions, and shared these with me, thus providing me with additional understanding. To me, this was valuable analysis provided by the participants themselves.

A second analysis was achieved by weaving together the stories, quotations from conversations, and field notes — arranged by themes — with the scholarly literature on each topic. This combination of what was seen and heard, with what has been published on these themes, provides the reader with an additional perspective.

A third component of understanding, the hermeneutical analysis, was reached through the writing of short original poems. As a researcher reviewing the materials, I thought about the essence of each story or observation. To communicate this essence in a concise and meaningful way, I wrote poetic interpretations. The poem is a way of communicating meaning without imposing extensive structure on the data. I agree with Ellis and Flaherty who say, "While any literary form imprisons lived experience...without some form or structure, it would be impossible to convey any experience."[221] Poetry provides succinct, yet dense, analysis. It is a means by which a researcher can communicate meaning received from the data. As van Manen suggests, poems are powerful means of sharing human experience because they do not require summaries. In his words, "The poem itself is the result.... To summarize a poem, to ask for the conclusion of it, would destroy the result.... The poem is the thing."[222] Poems are able to communicate both the details — including the tacit, unspoken — and the emotion of an experience within the limitations of words.

As a side note, as I have disseminated the findings of this study to nursing audiences, it is often the poems that people respond to in positive way. Many ask for copies of the poems because, in their words, "They speak to me," or "They touch my heart."

The thematic analysis is the most obvious dimension of the multi-layer analysis. The stories, transcripts, and journal entries regarding observations were analyzed thematically. The emergent themes from the data were revealed using a process Mitchell and Jones called "thematising."[223] Through reading and rereading the data sources, I eventually settled on the major themes that are within the data set. As part of the analysis process, Owen's suggestion for identifying themes by using three points of reference — recurrence of ideas within the data (ideas that have the same meaning but different wording), repetition (the existence of the same ideas using the same wording) and forcefulness (cues that reinforce a concept) — were employed.[224]

The final dimension of analysis is left to you, the reader. By reviewing the verbatim words of the participants and the analysis of the researcher, you will form your own insights about exemplary nursing making the analysis more complete and personalized.

This multi-part account, I feel, is close to the nurses' realities. It is designed to capture and communicate the sublime, unstructured, and non-verbal, as well as the more obvious themes.

## Trustworthiness

Qualitative research requires means for assuring standards of rigor. I believe that what readers need regarding trustworthiness is to know what I did as a researcher that would increase their trust in my ability as a researcher. Several actions were taken to ensure trustworthiness. For example, the nurse participants reviewed some of their own interview transcripts and field notes written on observations involving them. Written and verbal feedback and additional insights were offered by the nurses on these occasions. Two of the nurses reviewed drafts of the findings and stated they believed the insights represented their experiences.

Additionally, each method of data collection served as an opportunity to supplement the others. During the interviews, I was able to confirm my observations by sharing my findings and asking the nurses for clarification and further details. The interviews also provided a chance to discuss the analysis of the data as it was beginning to unfold. The narrative exchange netted stories that confirmed what I had been observing and hearing about during the interviews and what I had seen during the observation phase.

I also presented my preliminary findings to a small group of oncology nurses who were not involved in the study. These nurses commented that I was "getting the real picture" and "seeing exactly what was going on." The final findings have been disseminated to nurses across Canada and internationally. The feedback I have received from these audiences gives me confidence that this portrayal of exceptionally competent nursing is accurate.

Other strategies used in this study to increase data trustworthiness included keeping the nurses' comments verbatim and in context, tape-recording and transcribing interviews, using a research journal to record decision points in the research process, and using multiple data sources that confirmed one another. Prolonged engagement at the study site also enhanced credibility of the data. Data collection for this study took place over a period of 14 months, from May, 1992, to June, 1993.

This study is not meant to be replicated or generalized. It would be impossible to replicate because I studied a particular group of people at a particular time. Further studies of exceptional nurses would add to this body of knowledge; however, this study was designed to stand alone in the distinctive contribution it might make.

There are many considerations related to the use of self as a research instrument and the influence on data trustworthiness. Qualitative research requires the involvement of the researcher in this way. I was concerned initially that having been an oncology nurse for nine years prior to starting this project might negatively influence the quality of the study. Lipson notes that the quality of the data is influenced by the informant's perception of the researcher.[225] For example, the researcher's age, gender, culture, and profession may influence the amount, candidness, and honesty of the data. There was congruence been the participants and me on most of these factors. As a result of my experience as a cancer nurse, I was familiar with the role; yet, because I had not worked at the study site, I believe I was removed enough to be able to view it afresh.

Aguilar proposes that familiarity enhances ease of entry for the researcher because there is a common understanding of language, procedures, and experience. This can result in a more accurate account.[226] My comfort level on the unit, and consequently my ability to relate in a relaxed manner with staff and patients, was increased because I was familiar with the oncology milieu including the jargon, sights, smells, and emotion. To be a nurse, you need well-honed interviewing and observational skills which were directly transferable to my role as a researcher.

Another consideration in the use of self as a research instrument involves the researcher's own personal style, issues, values, and biases. Aamodt writes that the researcher's own ideas will pervade the research whether the researcher wills it or not, so therefore the best approach is assessment and acknowledgement of self prior to, and during, the research process.[227] Lipson observes that a beginning point is for the researcher to acknowledge these potential influences by describing his or her own background, giving the consumers of the research an understanding of where the researcher is "coming from" so they can make a judgment about the possible influence of the researcher's history.[228] Lipson contends that the researcher's biases should not be considered a limitation but should instead be capitalized on as a rich source of data and avenues of learning about the setting.[229] Further, Lipson emphasizes that researchers must have self-awareness to minimize the negative impact of their underlying personal landscape on the research process.[230] Interestingly, although self-awareness is important for good fieldwork, doing fieldwork also helps develop self-awareness as it brings you face to face with your own values. In an attempt to reveal some of my possible values and biases to readers, Chapter 2 includes some of my more poignant memories of working as an oncology nurse, plus reflections from my recent experience.

## Assumptions

The assumptions of this study are compatible with the philosophy of phenomenology. It is assumed that meaning is a central concept in that it mediates human interactions. People are not merely reactive organisms; rather, they think about, and are deliberate in, their actions. I assumed that the nurses shared their honest perspectives. Finally, I assume that the essence of a phenomenon can be understood, described, and shared—and, indeed, that there is such an entity as exceptional oncology nursing practice.

## Delimitations and limitations

One important boundary for this study is its focus on nurses who specialize in oncology. This can be viewed as a strength in that it concentrates the research on an in-depth investigation of this group. A further delimitation is related to the number of respondents; in this study, the sample was eight nurses. Perhaps it would have strengthened this study if I had spent more time with each nurse. Although the literature on qualitative research counsels that the researcher may conclude data gathering once the point of "data saturation" is reached, I am not convinced that data saturation ever really occurs. Within this particular study environment, there were many aspects of each interaction, and the elements were constantly changing. As long as I was exposed to the nurses who were meeting new patients daily, I was gaining enhanced — or perhaps new — understandings of exemplary nursing. However, given the reality that every study has to one day come to a formal end, data collection was limited to 14 months.

I realize there will always be explanations and ways of viewing these data other than those I have put forward in this book. As a researcher, I am limited by my abilities to perceive and communicate the meaning of experiences observed and discussed. I invite you to take what I have offered and to go beyond what I have done to venture alternative, or perhaps more insightful, understandings of exemplary oncology nursing. The data is presented in a way that it is available for remining.

## Ethical considerations

This research method carries with it many ethical considerations as I entered the nurses' worlds and sought to discover and report personal and intimate thoughts and experiences. It was a privilege to do so, and I made every effort not to abuse this. A fundamental principle guiding this research was that of beneficence, which encompasses the maxim: Above all, do no harm. With this in mind, I structured my design with the objective that no one concerned would be harmed or exploited, and so the potential of the benefits of the study would outweigh any risks. In consultation with the participants, we decided that the knowledge to be gained would have potential utility for many nurses and patients. The nurses also said that they would experience benefits such as increased self-awareness and enhanced self-esteem from participating and being labeled an exemplary nurse.

The informants and I discussed the possibility that participation in the study would change them and the way they provided care. We anticipated that reliving their meaningful nursing moments in the narrative exchange might cause them some personal distress.

To temper the potential harm, I made sufficient time to talk and debrief the nurses at various times. I was careful not to exploit the nurses' time by asking for too much. If I sensed that they needed, solitude, I gave them space — physically and psychologically. If I noticed that any nurse was uncomfortable being observed to the point that it might impact the quality of care she provided a patient, I simply left the scene. I did not want any patient to be denied an act of compassion because the nurse was uncomfortable with me watching the encounter.

Formal ethical approval for this study was granted by a university research ethics board. All participants in the study signed an informed consent form. All data collected were securely stored and identifiers removed. The original data were destroyed following analysis. While confidentially has been carefully guarded, total anonymity is never possible. The nurses who participated are known to each other and to me. I can link each participant with data associated with that participant. However, to facilitate anonymity to some extent, all examples have not been attributed to a specific respondent. Rather, sometimes comments, observations, and stories have been interwoven to provide an integrated picture of exemplary nursing practice.

I spent time preparing myself for field research, anticipating possible ethical situations that could arise and formulating what I thought would be appropriate responses. What would I do if I saw a nurse providing what I considered unsafe care? How would I respond if a patient in serious need asked me for help I couldn't give as a "volunteer"? What would my response be if a nurse I was observing asked for my help beyond my designated scope of practice or advice? By talking with the participants openly about my role before starting the study, these occasion were rare. My observer-as-participant stance also reduced the occurrence of these situations.

I also deliberated about how much I should disclose to informants about myself. My concern was that it was unjust to ask the nurses to share so much about themselves with me without disclosing something of my situation. Where was the point where sharing my own stories would increase the connection between us, and therefore candidness and depth of the interviews and narrative exchanges — and where would it interfere? Following the advice of Young and Tardif, I intentionally shared some of my own relevant experiences at appropriate moments in each relationship.[231]

Another ethical consideration was the need to be true to the nurses in the study — to record, interpret, and convey their feelings, thoughts, and actions accurately. I believe that, through ongoing verification with the nurses, accuracy was achieved. Reporting the findings in the nurses' own words and giving the nurses power to withhold any particular comment, story, or experience from the final research data was also important.

Finally, I deliberated whether ethically I had the right to even attempt to capture, understand, and communicate to others something so complex as human attitudes and behaviors. Would any attempt to discuss, describe, and share such actions and attitudes be so simplistic that a wrong would be done? Nursing is so intimate — should it be made public?

I anticipate that a variety of people can benefit from the findings of this study. Although my attempts to unravel the intricacies of exceptionally competent nursing practice and to transpose my understanding into words can be at best limited, I believe it was worthwhile to try.

This appendix described the design of the research study and the methodology on which it was based. Specific details of study participants, data collection procedures, and data analysis approaches were described. Techniques for maintaining data trustworthiness, the assumptions made, the delimitations and limitations of the study, and a discussion of ethical considerations were included.

# references

1. Kelly, P., and Crawford, H. 2008. *Nursing leadership and management: First Canadian edition* . Toronto: Nelson.

2. Perry, B. 2005. Core values brought to life: Exemplary nurses share their stories. *Nursing Standard* 20(7): 41–49.

3. Ibid.

4. Ibid.

5. LaRowe, K. 2005. Compassion fatigue: The heavy heart. http://www. compassion-fatigue.com/index.asp?PG=55 (accessed March 20, 2008), 21.

6. Schwam, K. 1998. The phenomenon of compassion fatigue in perioperative nursing. AORN *Journal*, 68:1–7.

7. Boychuk Duchscher, J., and Cowin, L. 2006. The new graduates' professional inheritance. *Nursing Outlook*, 54(3):152–158.

8. Jackson, C. 2004. Healing ourselves, healing others. *Holistic Nursing Practice*, 18(4):199–211.

9. Hagerty, J., Sherwood, P., Crighton, M., Song, M., and Happ, M. 2008. Conceptual challenges in the study of caregiver-care recipient relationships. *Nursing Research*, 57(5):367–372.

10. Scott, C. 2004. Nurses worried about erosion of the caring role. *British Journal of Nursing*, 13(7):348.

11. van Manen, M. 1990. *Researching lived experience: Human science for an action sensitive pedagogy*. London, ON: Althouse.

12. Ellis, C., and Flaherty, M. 1992. *Investigating subjectivity: Research on lived experience*. Newbury Park, CA: Sage, 3.

13. Milliken, T., Clements, P., & Tillman, H. 2007. The impact of stress management on nurse productivity and retention. *Nursing Economics,* 25(4):203–207.

14. Benner P, and Wrubel J. 1989. *The primacy of caring: Stress and coping in nursing*. London: Chapman/Hall.

15. Fagin, C., and Diers, D. 1983. Nursing as metaphor: Occasional notes. *New England Journal of Medicine*, 309:116.

16. Benner, P., and Wrubel, J. 1989.

17. Peplau, H. 1952. *Interpersonal relations in nursing.* NY: G.P. Putnam.

18. Mallison, M. 1987. How can you bear to be a nurse? *American Journal of Nursing*, 87(12):15–18.

19. Public Health Agency of Canada. 2004. http://www.phac-aspc.gc.ca/ publicat/lcd-pcd97/index-eng.php (accessed January 19, 2009).

20. Highfield, M. 1992.Spiritual health of oncology patients. *Cancer Nursing*, 15(1): 1–8.

21. Benner, P., and Wrubel, J. 1989, 8.

22. Glaser, B., and Strauss, A. 1968. *Awareness of dying.* Chicago: Aldine.

23. Benner, P., and Wrubel, J. 1989, 256.

24. Gauthier, D. 2008. Challenges and opportunities: Communication near the end of life. *Medsurg Nursing,* 17(5): 291–297.

25. Blondis, M., and Jackson, B. 1982. *Nonverbal communication with patients: Back to the human touch* (2nd ed.). NY: Wiley.

26. Armstrong, P. 2008. Requiem for the sounds of silence. *Canadian Medical Association Journal,* 178(8):1104.

27. Ibid.

28. Blondis, M., and Jackson, B. 1982, 42.

29. Bottorff, J. 1991. The lived experience of being comforted by a nurse. *Phenomenology and pedagogy,* 9:237–252.

30. Clayton, C., Murray, J., Horner, S., and Grene, P. 1991. Connecting: A catalyst for caring. In P. Chinn (Ed.), *An anthology of caring.* NY: National League for Nursing.

31. Watson, J. 1989. Human caring and suffering: A subjective model for health services. In J. Watson and R. Taylor (Eds.), *They shall not hurt: Human suffering and human caring* . Boulder, CO: Colorado Associated University.

32. Ibid., 129.

33. Marcel, G. 1969. *The philosophy of existence* . Freeport, NY: Books University, 25–26.

34. Ibid.

35. Green-Hernandez, C. 1991. A phenomenological investigation of caring as a lived experience in nursing. In P. Chinn (Ed.), *An anthology of caring.* NY: National League for Nursing, 120.

36. Watson, J. 1989.

37. Bottorff, J. 1991, 244–245.

38. O'Banion, T., and O'Connell, A. (1970). *The shared journey: An introduction to encounter.* Englewood Cliffs, NJ: Prentice-Hall, 161.

39. Blondis, M., and Jackson, B. 1982, viii.

40. Roberts, L., and Bucksey, S. 2007. Communicating with patients: What happens in practice? *Physical Therapy,* 87(5): 586–595.

41. Ibid.

42. Ibid.

43. Blondis, M., and Jackson, B. 1982, 170.

44. Watson, J. 1989.

45. Taylor, C. 1991. On the way to teaching as letting learn. *Phenomenology and Pedagogy,* 9:351–355, 353.

46. Caputo, J. 1978. *The mystical element in Heidegger's thought.* Athens: Oberlin, 117.

47. Naisbitt, J. 1982. *Megatrends: Ten new directions transforming our lives*. NY: Warner, 40.

48. Tough, J. 1989. *The psychophysiological effects of back massage in elderly institutionalized patients*. Master's thesis, University of Alberta, Edmonton, AB, 120.

49. Watson, J. 1989, 130.

50. Ryan, K. 2008. The inhospitable hospital: No peace, no quiet. *RNformation*, 17(4):1.

51. Sims, S. 1986. Slow stroke back massage for cancer patients. *Nursing Times*, 82(13): 47–50.

52. Montagu, A. 1986. *Touching: The human significance of skin* (3rd ed.). NY: Harper/Row.

53. Bottorff, J. 1991. A methodological review and evaluation of research on nurse-patient touch. In P. Chinn (Ed.), *An anthology of caring*. NY: National League for Nursing.

54. Barraja-Rohan, A. 2000. Teaching conversation and sociocultural norms with conversation analysis. In Liddicoat, A.J., Crozet, C. (Eds.). *Teaching languages, teaching cultures*. Melbourne: Language Australia.

55. Benner, P. 1984. *From novice to expert: Excellence and power in clinical nursing practice*. Melno Park, CA: Addison-Wesley, 165.

56. Routasalo P. 1996. Non-necessary touch in the nursing care of elderly people. *Journal of Advanced Nursing*, 23:904–911.

57. Ibid.

58. Chang, S. 2001. Nursing theory and concept development or analysis. *Journal of Advanced Nursing*, 33(6):820–827.

59. Watson, J. 1989, 129.

60. Langer-Albert, M., and Short, S. 1994. Nutritional intake, use of touch and verbal cuing. *Journal of Gerontological Nursing* 20:36–40.

61. Montagu, A. 1986, 282.

62. Gadow, S. 1984. Touch and technology: Two paradigms of patient care. *Journal of Religion and Health*, 23:63–69.

63. Benner, P. 1984, 64.

64. Watson, J. 1985. Human caring and suffering: A subjective model for health services. In J. Watson and R. Taylor (Eds.), *They shall not hurt: Human suffering and human caring*. Boulder, CO: Colorado Associated University, 129.

65. Barraja-Rohan, A. 2000.

66. Montagu, A. 1986, 125.

67. Estabrooks, C., and Morse, J. 1992. Toward a theory of touch: The touching process and acquiring a touch style. *Journal of Advanced Nursing* 17:448–456.

68. Bottorff, J. 1991.
69. Routasalo P. 1996.
70. Estabrooks, C., and Morse, J. 1992.
71. Routasalo, P. 1996.
72. Watson, J. 1985.
73. Barraja-Rohan, A. 2000.
74. Montagu, A. 1986, 133.
75. Davidhizar, R., and Giger, J. 1997. When touch is not the best approach. *Journal of Clinical Nursing* 6: 203–206.
76. Caris-Verhallen, W., Kerkstra, A., and Bensing, J. 1999. Non-verbal behaviour in nurse-elderly patient communication. *Journal of Advanced Nursing*, 29(4): 808–818.
77. Montagu, A. 1986.
78. Routasalo P. 1996.
79. Bartenieff, I., and Lewis, D. 1980. *Body movement: Coping with the environment.* NY: Gordon/Breach.
80. Ibid., 396.
81. Montagu, A. 1986.
82. Estabrooks, C., and Morse, J. 1992.
83. Davidhizar, R., and Giger, J. 1997.
84. Watson, J. 1989.
85. Chang, S. 2001.
86. Montagu, A. 1986, 264.
87. Ibid., 264.
88. Bottorff, J. 1992. *Nurse-patient interaction: Observations of touch.* Doctoral dissertation, University of Alberta, Edmonton, AB.
89. Estabrooks, C. 1987. *Touching behaviors of ICU nurses.* Master's thesis, University of Alberta, Edmonton, AB.
90. Montagu, A. 1986, 124.
91. Levine, S. 1987. *Healing into life and death.* Garden City, NJ: Doubleday.
92. Bartenieff, I., and Lewis, D. 1980, 287.
93. Ibid.
94. Bottorff, J. 1992, 287.
95. Hagen, C. 1989. *Inspirited-dispirited touch: A phenomenological investigation.* Doctoral dissertation, Texas Women's University.
96. Watson, J. 1989.
97. Bottorff, J. 1992.
98. Montagu, A. 1986, 270.
99. Barraja-Rohan, A. 2000, 133.
100. Morse, J. 1983. An ethnoscientific analysis of comfort: A preliminary investigation. *Nursing Papers*, 15(1):6–19, 16.

101. Ibid.

102. Benner, P. 1984, 63.

103. Montagu, A. 1986, 284.

104. Watson, J. 1989, 23.

105. Chang, S. 2001.

106. Watson, J. 1989, 22.

107. The Bible: King James Version. http://etext.virginia.edu/kjv.browse.html (accessed January 21, 2009).

108. Pasquali, E. 1990. Learning to laugh: Humor as therapy. Journal of Psychosocial Nursing, 28:31–35.

109. Parfitt, J. 1990. Humorous preoperative teaching. American Operating Room Nurses Journal, 52:114–120.

110. Gaberson, K. 1991. The effect of humorous distraction on preoperative anxiety. American Operating Room Nurses Journal, 54:1258–1263.

111. Erdman, L. 1991. Laughter therapy for patients with cancer. Oncology Nursing Forum, 18:1359–1363.

112. Thomas, J. 1983. Extending oneself: Humor as a medium in social studies education. Master's thesis. University of Alberta, Edmonton, AB.

113. Benner, P., and Wrubel, J. 1989, 19.

114. Robinson, V. 1991. Humor and the health professions. Thorofare, NJ: Slack.

115. Thomas, J. 1983.

116. Astedt-Kurki, P., and Liukkonen, A. 1994. Humor in nursing. Journal of Advanced Nursing, 20(1):183–191.

117. Hunt, A. 1993. Humor as a nursing intervention. Cancer Nursing, 16(1):34–39, 35.

118. Baughman, M. 1974. Baughman's handbook of humor in education. West Nyack, NY: Parker, 52.

119. Thomas, J. 1983.

120. Lefcourt, H., and Martin, R. 1986. Humor and life stress. NY: Springer-Verlag, 58.

121. Leacock, S. 1938. Humour and humanity: An introduction to the study of humour. NY: Henry Holt.

122. Olsson, H., Backe, H., Sorensen, S., and Kock, M. 2002. The essence of humour and its effects and functions: a qualitative study. Journal of Nursing Management, 10(1):21–26.

123. Benner, P., and Wrubel, J. 1989, 19.

124. Dean, R., and Major, J. 2008. The relational humor inventory: Functions of humor in close relationships. Journal of Clinical Nursing, 17(8):1088–1095.

125. Ibid., 1088.

126. McDougall, W. 1963. An instinct of laughter: An introduction to social psychology. NY: Barnes/Noble, 135.

127.  Baughman, M. 1974, 52.
128.  Yura H., and Walsh M. 1988. *The nursing process*, (5th ed.). East Norwalk, CT: Appleton & Lange.
129.  Hunt, A. 1993.
130.  Ibid., 34.
131.  Pasquali, E. 1990.
132.  Blondis, M., and Jackson, B. 1982, 189.
133.  Leacock, S. 1938.
134.  Moody, R. 1978. *Laugh after laughter: The healing power of humor.* Jacksonville, FL: Headwaters, 120.
135.  Dean, R., and Major, J. 2008.
136.  De Koning, E., and Weiss, R. 2002. From critical care to comfort care: The sustaining value of humour. *American Journal of Family Therapy*, 30:1–18.
137.  Baughman, M. 1974.
138.  Dean, R., and Major, J. 2008.
139.  Ibid.
140.  Ibid.
141.  Baughman, M. 1974, 61.
142.  De Koning, E., and Weiss, R. 2002.
143.  Baughman, M. 1974, 56.
144.  Bradford, A. 1964. The place of humor in teaching. *Peabody Journal of Education*, 42(2): 67–70, 70.
145.  Gruner, C. 1978. *Understanding laughter: The workings of wit and humor.* Chicago: Nelson-Hall, 1.
146.  Baughman, M. 1974, 52.
147.  Spiegel, K. 1972. Early conceptions of humor: Varieties and issues. In J. Goldstein & P. McGhee (Eds.), *The psychology of humor: Theoretical perspectives.* NY: Academic Press, 7.
148.  Gelazis, R. 1991. Creative strategies for teaching care. In M. Leininger and D. Gaut (Eds.), *Caring: The compassionate healer.* NY: National League for Nursing.
149.  Hunt, A. 1993, 37.
150.  Gelazis, R. 1991, 259.
151.  Leacock, S. 1938, 8.
152.  Benner, P., and Wrubel, J. 1989, 19.
153.  Leacock, S. 1938, 8.
154.  Clayton, C., Murray, J., Horner, S., and Grene, P. 1991, 155.
155.  Frankl, V. 1959. *Man's search for meaning.* Boston, MA: Beacon Hill.
156.  Burke, M. 1985. The personal and professional journey of James B. MacDonald. *Journal of Curriculum Theorizing*, 6(3):84–119, 95.
157.  Levine, S. 1987, 77.

158. Benner, P. 1984, 209.

159. McHutchion, E. 1987. *The family perspective on dying at home.* Doctoral dissertation, University of Alberta, Edmonton, AB, 320.

160. O'Banion, T., and O'Connell, A. 1970, 160.

161. Watson, J. 1989, 132.

162. Watson, J. 1985, 43.

163. Ibid., 58.

164. Ibid., 59.

165. Ibid., 160.

166. O'Banion, T., and O'Connell, A. 1970.

167. Wiedenbach, E. 1964. *Clinical nursing: A helping art.* NY: Springer.

168. Watson, J. 1989.

169. Ibid., 131.

170. O'Banion, T., and O'Connell, A. 1970, 7.

171. Eakes, G. 1993. The emotional impact of living with cancer. *Oncology Nursing Forum,* 20(9):13–35.

172. O'Banion, T., and O'Connell, A. 1970.

173. Askinazi, A. 2004. Caring about caring. *Nursing Forum,* 39(2):33–36.

174. Ibid.

175. Hagerty, B., and Patusky, K. 2003. Reconceptualizing the nurse-patient relationship. *Journal of Nursing Scholarship,* 31(2):145–150.

176. Levine, S. 1987, 17.

177. Perry, B. 2009. Achieving professional fulfillment as a palliative care nurse. *Journal of Hospice and Palliative Nursing,* 11(2):109–118.

178. Macnee, C., and McCabe, S. 2008. *Understanding nursing research: Reading and using research in evidence-based practice* (2$^{nd}$ ed.). New York: Lippincott Williams & Wilkins.

179. Benner, P., and Wrubel, J. 1989.

180. Loiselle, C., and Profetto-McGrath, J. 2004. *Canadian essentials of nursing research.* NY: Lippincott Williams & Wilkins.

181. Ibid.

182. Ibid.

183. van Manen, M. 1990.

184. Wilson, H. & Hutchinson, S. 1991.Triangulation of qualitative methods: Heideggerian hermeneutics and grounded theory. *Qualitative Health Researcher,* 1(2):263–276.

185. van Manen, M. 1990, 38.

186. Laverty, S. 2003. Hermeneutic phenomenology and phenomenology: A comparison of historical and methodological considerations. *International Journal of Qualitative Methods,* 2(3). http://www.ualberta.ca/~iiqm/ backissues/2_3final/pdf/laverty.pdf (accessed January 21, 2009).

187. Gaut, D. 1981. A philosophical method to study phenomena. In M. Leininger (Ed.), *Qualitative research methods in nursing*. NY: Grune/ Stratton.

188. Merleau-Ponty, M. 1962. *The phenomenology of perception*. London: Routledge & Kegan, 39.

189. van Manen, M. 1990, 10.

190. Ibid., 36.

191. Ibid., 9.

192. Ibid., 7.

193. Heidegger, M. 1962. *Being and time*. NY: Harper/Row.

194. van Manen, M. 1990, 12.

195. Ibid., 18.

196. Mérleau-Ponty, M. 1962.

197. Gadamer, H. 1975. *Truth and method*. NY: Seaburg.

198. van Manen, M. 1990, 34.

199. Benner, P., and Wrubel, J. 1989.

200. Morse, J. (Ed.). 1991. *Qualitative nursing research: A contemporary dialogue*, Newbury Park, CA: Sage.

201. Ibid.

202. Benner, P. 1984.

203. Wright, S., and Carrese, J. 2002. Excellence in role modeling: Insight and perspectives from the pros. *Canadian Medical Association Journal*, 167(6): 638–643.

204. Benner, P., and Wrubel, J. 1989.

205. Pearsall, M. 1965. Participant observation as role and method in behavioral research. *Nursing Research*, 14(1):37–42.

206. Ibid.

207. Levine, S. 1987.

208. Polit, D., and Hungler, B. 2001. *Essentials of nursing research: Methods, appraisal and utilization* (5th ed.). New York: Lippincott Williams & Wilkins, 325.

209. Benner, P. 1984.

210. Ellis, C., and Flaherty, M. 1992.

211. Ibid., 6.

212. Polit, D., and Hungler, B. 2001, 329.

213. Anderson, J. 1991.The phenomenological perspective. In J. Morse (Ed.), *Qualitative nursing research: A contemporary dialogue*. Newbury Park, CA: Sage, 35.

214. van Manen, M. 1990, 34.

215. Ibid., 32.

216. Ibid., 32.

217. Anderson, J. 1991.

218. Oiler, C. 1986. Phenomenology: The method. In P. Munhall and C. Oiler (Eds.), *Nursing research: A qualitative perspective.* Norwalk, CT: Appleton-Century-Crofts.

219. Ibid., 2.

220. Ibid.

221. Ellis, C., and Flaherty, M. 1992, 123.

222. van Manen, M. 1990, 13.

223. Mitchell, T., and Jones, S. 2004. Leading and co-ordinating a multi-nurse researcher project. *Nurse Researcher,* 12(2): 42–56.

224. Owen, W. 2002 Interpretative themes in relational communication. *Quarterly Journal of Speech,* 70:274–287.

225. Lipson, J. 1991.The use of self in ethnographic research. In J. Morse (Ed.), *Qualitative nursing research: A contemporary dialogue.* Newbury Park, CA: Sage.

226. Aguilar, J. 1981. Insider research: An ethnography of a debate. In D. Messerschmidt (Ed.), *Anthropologist in North America.* Cambridge: Cambridge University Press.

227. Aamodt, A. 1991. Ethnography and epistemology: Generating nursing knowledge. In J. Morse (Ed.), *Qualitative nursing research: A contemporary dialogue.* Newbury Park, CA: Sage.

228. Lipson, J. 1991.

229. Ibid.

230. Ibid.

231. Young, B., and Tardif, C. 1992. Interviewing: Two sides of the story. *Qualitative Studies in Education,* 5(2):135–145.